Preface

D0584091

Public health requires everyone to work to improve health and tackle inequalities in health. The 2004 NHS Improvement Plan says: 'In taking forward the public health agenda there is a need to strengthen the public health capacity … to ensure that the right people, skills and approaches are in place both in the NHS and in partner agencies to make sure improvement, health protection and health inequalities are actively pursued.'

Over recent years there has been a growing recognition that public health is not solely the domain and responsibility of public health departments and specialist public health nurses. There is increasing awareness of the need to build and strengthen public health knowledge, capability and capacity throughout the health-care workforce. Many nurses and other health-care practitioners are often keen to address issues of public health but don't always know where to start. This book aims to address this issue and demonstrate that, regardless of where you work or the patients or clients you are working with, there is real potential to view public health as a constant and central tenet of professional health-care practice. Indeed we believe it is vital that you do.

The book is intended to help nurses and other health-care practitioners learn and apply the knowledge and skills of public health to their own area of practice. Each chapter has a range of features designed to help you. As some of the terms may well be unfamiliar, we define key words as we go along. Each chapter begins with its learning outcomes and ends with a rapid recap to review what you've learned. Some chapters have summaries of key points. Reflective activities encourage you to reflect on your current practice, and over-to-you features invite you to look at new ideas and the potential for public health practice. Many of these activities arise from real-life situations. The text is interspersed with case studies and the words of working health professionals. Look out for top tips to improve your practice. Public health is a large field of study and relies on a growing evidence base. Key references are listed at the end of every chapter, but other important references are given in the evidence base feature dotted throughout the text. Some references are to websites, and the URLs for these are available on the publisher's website (www.nelsonthornes.com).

Chapter 1 outlines the historical context of public health and the impact of policy on the practice of public health. All public health practitioners need a thorough understanding of the roots of public health and its policy drivers. Chapter 1 pays attention to health inequalities as much of the recent government policy is driven by the need to deliver better outcomes for the poorest in our communities. Chapter 2 sets out the principles and key concepts of public health practice. It will help familiarise you with the language and terminology of public health and with some ways of working. Chapter 3 will help you think about how to apply principles of public health practice to your own area of work. It includes a model for practice based on the 10 key areas of public health practice. Although many of its examples refer to nursing, we hope that much of the material is applicable to any area of health-care practice and to anyone wishing to work in the field of public health.

We wanted our book to be a practical guide, so Chapters 4 to 8 are a step-by-step approach to developing your public health practice. The cornerstone of public health practice is a health needs assessment (HNA) of the community you work with. Chapters 4 and 5 show you how to plan an HNA, gather data and appraise the evidence. Chapter 6 considers how to decide which intervention is most appropriate and focuses primarily on health promotion. It gives a critical review of the available models. This will help you decide on the best approaches to adapt and adopt in your work. Chapter 7 looks at the challenges of building relationships on solid foundations. Public health is not a lone endeavour; it requires multiple perspectives, multiple approaches and robust partnerships. Chapter 8 is on evaluation. It is essential to evaluate public health initiatives by process, outcome and impact. The body of public health evidence on what works is still in its infancy and needs to be firmly established by rigorous evaluation.

Chapter 9 describes developments in public health practice at home and abroad. Written from the perspective of public health nurses, it gives an insight into the highs and lows found in practice. We hope these examples inspire you to embrace public health practice in your own work. Collectively, we believe, practitioners can make a difference to the health of the public. Throughout the book we have used the term 'community' in its broadest sense to mean any group, population or neighbourhood. A multitude of terms are used in policy and practice to describe the people we work with – patients, clients, consumers and service users – yet none seems entirely satisfactory. In the interests of consistency, we have chosen 'patient' and 'client' as they are the terms most frequently used by nurses, community nurses and health-care practitioners and we think they will be the largest share of our readers.

1
Public health policy

Ivy O'Neil

Learning outcomes

By the end of this chapter you should be able to:

★ Understand the context of public health and public health policy in Britain

★ Identify the key milestones in public health development

★ Outline the implications of public health policy development for nursing and health-care practice.

⚡️🔑 *Keywords*
....

Public health

Smith and Jacobson (1988) stated that public health 'involves the promotion of health, the prevention of disease, the treatment of illness, the care of those who are disabled, and the continuous development of the technical and social means for the pursuit of these objectives'. Acheson (1988, p.16) defines 'public health' as 'the art and science of preventing disease, prolonging life, promoting, protecting and improving health and well-being through the organised efforts of society'

Introduction

Public health has always been important in health care and successive governments have tried to address and improve the health of the public in different ways. Since the current Labour government came to power in 1997 and published the first public health White Paper, *Saving Lives: Our Healthier Nation* (Department of Health 1999a), there has been a sharp increase in awareness of the importance of public health. The Acheson Report (Acheson 1998) reignited concerns about fundamental inequalities in health – that the worst off in society are more ill and die earlier. This led to the development of many policies (Department of Health 1999a, 2001a, 2001b, 2001c, 2004a, 2004b, 2004c) emphasising the need for rigorous strategies to improve the health of the population.

This chapter explores the origins and development of public health and concentrates on the government's policies and strategies for improving health and reducing health inequalities. It is crucial that nurses and others wishing to work in the field of public health, in whatever capacity, have an awareness of the roots of public health theory and practice plus a thorough understanding of current public health policies at local and national levels.

Health trends and health policy

Policy outlines a set of objectives and rules that guide the activities of an organisation or an administration (Koelen and Van den Ban 2004). In public health terms, it defines priorities and scope for action in response to health needs. It helps set priorities in health-care provision and gives a framework for health-care delivery. It shapes and is shaped by key values and beliefs about health care and supports strategic planning and development. It also establishes systems for allocating resources and creates a means of tackling health inequalities.

The top five common causes of death in the UK are circulatory disease, cancer, respiratory disease, infectious disease, and injury and poisoning. Circulatory disease is the most common and cancer the second most common (Office for National Statistics 2006). Mortality rates by cause of death vary with age and sex (Figures 1.1 and 1.2). For young people and men aged 30–44 the most common cause of death is injury and poisoning. For women aged 30–65 it is cancer. For men and women aged 65–84 it is circulatory disease followed by respiratory diseases and cancers. Yet it is known that 25 per cent of all cancers and 30 per cent of coronary heart disease are preventable through public health measures (Wanless 2002).

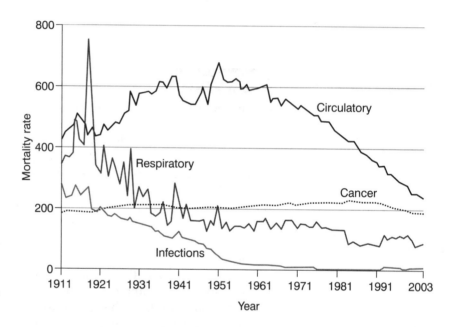

Figure 1.1 England and Wales: age-standardised mortality rates per 100,000 people for selected broad disease groups, 1911–2003. Reprinted with permission from the Office for National Statistics

○━π **Keywords**

Health promotion
The World Health Organization defined health promotion as the process of enabling people to increase control over their health and to improve their health (WHO 1984). It includes health education as well as policy development, engaging, enabling and empowering the people within the community in an attempt to address the wider environmental and social issues that adversely affect people's health

Traditionally, public health is about the prevention of disease but the pattern of disease has changed over time. Many infectious diseases that once caused death and devastation, such as cholera and smallpox, have been brought under control and are no longer considered a threat. But new problems have emerged, such as avian flu and HIV/AIDS, and other diseases are making a comeback, such as tuberculosis. At the top of today's health-care agenda are illnesses caused by our modern lifestyle: obesity leads to circulatory disease and diabetes; smoking leads to lung cancer; alcohol misuse leads to liver cirrhosis; complex societal factors lead to stress, depression and other mental health problems. Nowadays, public health covers a much broader range of issues and problems, although disease prevention is still seen as central to public health activity. **Health promotion** is growing rapidly and there is a strong emphasis on the role of the government in protecting people through healthy public policies. Public health involves a collective responsibility, the involvement of the state and the individual's responsibility.

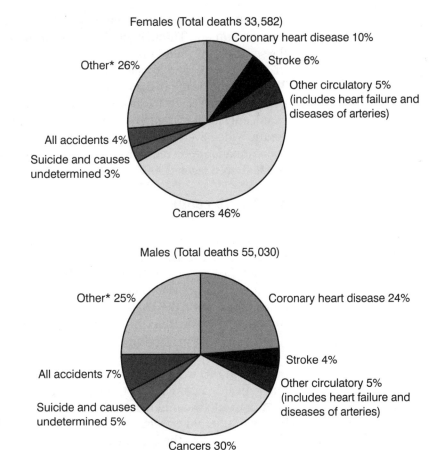

Figure 1.2 Causes of death among males and females. Reprinted, with permission, from Department of Health (1999a)
*This category includes causes of death other than those identified as priority areas (DH 1999a) and deaths occurring at ages under 28 days, which are included in the totals but are not allocated to a specific cause of death

Reflective activity

Think about your workplace. What are the most common conditions of patients, clients or service users you care for? Discuss them with your colleagues? How have they changed in recent years?

Historical perspective

Origins of public health

Public health has a long history and attempts to promote health and prevent disease were made even by the earliest civilisations (Rosen 1993). The Egyptians and the Incas understood the importance of urban planning and sanitation. They imposed rules to promote good diet and hygiene among the people. The Romans built aqueducts, public baths and sewage systems and purified their water supplies to prevent the outbreak of epidemics. This demonstrates an early understanding of the link between ill health and the environment. Throughout history, people have made efforts to prevent the spread of infectious disease. During the fourteenth century, harsh treatments were used to isolate and protect people from the Black Death. To protect the health of the rest of the population, people with leprosy were banished from society to isolated colonies (Rosen 1993). However, public health only really started to emerge at the beginning of the nineteenth century when overcrowded accommodation, inadequate ventilation and poor sanitation were recognised as important issues for the health of the population (Baggott 2000).

Nineteenth century

In the early part of the nineteenth century, large parts of England had become industrialised and living and working conditions were poor and lacked even basic sanitation. There were regular outbreaks of diseases such as cholera, tuberculosis and typhoid. Some industrial cities had mortality rates of over 40 per 1,000 in the adult population and over half of all children died before age 5. This was an issue not only for the working classes but also for the factory owners and entrepreneurs who relied on a healthy workforce. Indeed the realisation that the health of the most deprived members of society had to be of concern to the population as a whole was a strong factor in providing the impetus for public health action at that time (Orme *et al.* 2003).

As a result, the mid to late nineteenth century was characterised by environmental change and the Victorian sanitary revolution. Edwin Chadwick, the secretary of the Poor Law Commission, in his report on the sanitary conditions of the labouring population of Great Britain (Chadwick 1842, cited in Baggott 2000) recognised the link between environment and disease. The government responded and the first Public Health Act was introduced in 1848. It aimed to improve environmental health and reduce death and disease by improving living conditions, installing water supplies and sewage systems (Ham 2004). It could be argued that these reforms, together with major legislation governing factories and mines, led to greater improvements in the population's health than any subsequent advances in medical interventions or developments in the NHS (Baggott 2000).

Personal health and hygiene were also emphasised. A number of voluntary organisations emerged, such as the Ladies Sanitary Reform Movement. They were intent on improving not only the hygiene of the urban poor, but also their moral and social welfare as high levels of alcohol consumption and debauchery added to the problems in the inner cities.

During the cholera epidemic of 1854, John Snow discovered that the water supply from a particular pump in Broadgate, London, was associated with the outbreak. This was the beginning of evidence-based public health practice. Snow was able to map reported cases and identify the source of the disease. He observed events and spent time with

○━π Keywords

Epidemiology
Epidemiology is the study of the distribution, frequency and determinants of health and disease in the population. It is the basic science that underpins public health. It describes the health of groups of people, explains patterns of health and disease, evaluates the effectiveness and efficiency of health services and treatments, and provides evidence for health policy and health-care planning (Health Development Agency 2004)

the people to find out about their habits and practices. This provided compelling evidence of the cause of cholera, preceding the identification of the disease agent (*Vibrio cholerae*) by some 30 years. This discovery contributed to the formulation of germ theory and was subsequently seen as a classic example of **epidemiology** (Chapters 4 and 5). So began the influence of the medical profession in public health.

Early twentieth century

The early twentieth century, thought by some to be the golden age for public health (Holland and Stewart 1998), predominantly focused on personal preventive measures. In many ways this represented a further step in the medicalisation of public health and a fundamental shift in focus from the general population toward specific vulnerable groups and individuals. During the Boer War, the poor physical condition of the army recruits had raised concerns about the state of the population's general health. This was largely attributed to environmental and social influences on health. A range of measures was called for and emphasis was placed on maternal and child welfare services. Immunisation, screening in the form of school medical inspections and hygiene advice were essential components of the approach to public health at that time, which was essentially paternalistic (Orme *et al.* 2003). In 1919 the Ministry for Health was formed and given statutory responsibility for taking steps to coordinate measures conducive to the health of the people: environmental health, water supply and sanitation, maternal and child welfare services, the national health insurance scheme and the Poor Law.

This era was closely followed by a period characterised by developments in therapeutic interventions made possible by the discovery of antibiotic therapy. Public health became dominated by medical treatments, particularly those associated with new technology. Preventive public health work, although not forgotten, was certainly marginalised during this period.

Creation of the NHS

In the 1940s the British Medical Association recommended extending state involvement in health services. The 1942 Beveridge Report on social insurance and allied services stated that social and economic inequality was the cause of many health-related problems. Pressure from trade unions to provide better conditions for people who had contributed to the war effort added to the impetus. As a result, in 1948 the National Health Service was born, designed to deliver a comprehensive, free and accessible service with a clear distinction between services for ill health and preventive services. It emphasised the health of the public as a national priority and responsibility. This was regarded by many as a major public health achievement. Although others have since been critical, considering it to be an illness service not a health service.

During this time the responsibility for public health remained with the local authority, where a medical officer of health led a team of public health practitioners, including environmental health officers, health visitors and welfare officers dealing with population health issues. In 1974 the NHS underwent a radical reorganisation and the services were removed from local authorities to the NHS. Klein (1980) argued that Britain then had health services with no health policies. A limited number of measures were introduced, such as the child immunisation programme, the Clean Air Act 1956 and the Road Safety Act 1967, which made the speed limit 70 miles per hour (112 kph) and implemented more stringent drink-driving laws.

The 'new' public health era

In the early 1970s, the prevailing medical model of public health was becoming widely criticised as it was thought by some to focus on narrow scientific medical explanations for disease while ignoring far more complex health-harming social issues. The publication of the Lalonde Report in Canada in 1974 affirmed this perspective and marked the beginning of a new era in public health (Lalonde 1974). In 1977 the World Health Organization (WHO) committed itself to the principles of health for all, or HFA 2000, and endorsed the view that inequality was politically, socially and economically unacceptable. The HFA 2000 principles were founded on equity and also emphasised the need for collaborative actions to promote health. The first conference for promoting the health of the public was organised by WHO in 1986. This led to the Ottawa Charter that recommended 38 targets for achieving HFA (WHO 1986).

A second conference in Adelaide in 1988 focused on the importance of healthy public policies (WHO 1988). Health promotion became an important strategy in improving the health of the public. The third conference in Sweden in 1991 focused on supportive environments for better health and the development of health promotion in schools, hospitals and workplaces (WHO 1991). The United Nations Conference on Environment and Development (UNCED) in Brazil published the Agenda 21 strategies, which emphasised the importance of controlling communicable diseases, protecting vulnerable groups, and reducing health risk caused by pollution and excessive energy consumption and waste (United Nations 1993). The Jakarta Declaration on leading health promotion into the twenty-first century (WHO 1997) was developed at the fourth conference on health promotion. It emphasised the comprehensive approaches to health promotion and the importance of partnership involving the private sector in an active way. The concern for equity is at the core of health promotion which runs through the previous conferences. The fifth conference, held in Mexico in 2000, stated that health promotion is a fundamental component in public policies in the pursuit of equity and health for all (WHO 2000). It reinstated the relevance of health promotion; focus on the determinants of health and bridging the equity gap. The Bangkok Charter was published after the sixth Global Conference held in Thailand, 2005. In order to manage the challenges and opportunities of globalisation, collaboration and engagement of all sectors in the society is needed to promote the health of the people (Tang *et al.* 2006).

Conservative government

Despite the background of international developments and the publication of the Black Report on inequalities in Britain's health (Black *et al.* 1980), the Conservative government of the time was opposed to any central strategy for public health. In accordance with its own political ideology, it favoured two main approaches: individual responsibility and managerialism in public services. Firstly, emphasis was placed on changing the lifestyle of the individual. Indeed the leader of the government, Margaret Thatcher, asserted that 'society does not exist' (Shaw 1994). Prevention activities mainly used medical approaches to prevent disease and employed screening techniques to detect early disease such as cervical and breast cancer.

Treating ill health and hospital care were still important aspects of the health service. The focus was on surgery and high technology, which required a large amount of resources. Secondly, the government was keen to make the NHS more managerially competitive – a better business. Cost-effectiveness, but really cost minimisation, was a major feature in the management of health services. Policies on improving the health of the people were restrictive. The focus on competition and the internal health-care markets were not conducive to holistic and collaborative approaches. During the 1980s there was a lack of government policy direction and funding in public health; progress was understandably disappointing.

Nevertheless, throughout the 1990s, the promotion of health became more important. Many public health issues were raised because of the increased activities of pressure groups. *The Health of the Nation* (Department of Health 1992) was an important but contentious landmark for the Conservative government in health care and public health. Critics said that the targets were disease oriented, focusing on the medical model of health rather than a social perspective of health, ignoring the wider determinants of health. Prevention was less important than reducing waiting lists. Again the policies reflected the right-wing ideology of individualism. The socio-economic causes of ill health and the inequality of social deprivation were seen as irrelevant. Policies related more to the prevention of specific diseases rather than to the promotion of health and the tackling of poverty.

🔑 Keywords

Community
Community has several meanings. A community can be the geographical or physical area where a person lives, but it can also be a place of education (school, college), a place of work (factory, office, hospital), a place of worship (mosque, church, synagogue), or a place of social or sports activity (working men's club, luncheon club, football club). It can encompass a combination of factors, such as a group of older, Asian men with diabetes

🔑 Keywords

Efficiency
Concerned with how goals have been achieved compared with other ways of achieving them

🔑 Keywords

National Service Frameworks
Long-term strategies for improving specific areas of care. They identify key interventions and set standards and measurable goals within set timeframes

New Labour government

In fulfilling its election promise to safeguard and improve the NHS, a whole wave of policies came forth from the Department of Health in the early years of the New Labour government. The internal market favoured by the previous administration was immediately abolished and *The New NHS, Modern, Dependable* (Department of Health 1997) paved the way for the modernisation of the NHS. It stated the three developments that symbolised the new NHS:

- **at home** – better advice and information services
- **in the community** – swift advice and treatment, collaboration between departments, quicker results and better computer links
- **in hospital** – prompt access to specialist services, particularly for cancer.

Here are the six principles of the NHS:

- renewing the NHS as a genuinely national service
- delivery of health care is a local responsibility
- partnership with local authority and provision of patient-centred care
- driving **efficiency** by a more rigorous approach to performance
- focus on quality of care so that excellence is the norm
- rebuilding public confidence in the NHS as a public service.

In public health there was something of a renaissance. After the general election, the first minister for public health was appointed, demonstrating the government's commitment to tackling inequalities in health and public health issues. A greater emphasis was placed on the social, economic and environmental factors that influence health and this was seen as a significant step forward by commentators at the time: 'The re-engagement of public health practitioners with the social and environmental determinants of health is both long overdue and welcome' (Hunter 1999, p.12).

There was a commitment to social reforms such as housing, education and transport. The priorities were on reducing waiting lists, improving breast cancer services, reducing smoking-related illness, and tackling postcode prescribing (Department of Health 1999a). The health service became less driven by competition and more focused on health – a national contract for better health based on partnership and driven by performance. The provision of quality services was and remains the main agenda. Service standards would be set through the National Institute for Health and Clinical Excellence (NICE) and the **National Service Frameworks** (NSFs) would set out specific standards for services and recommend best practice underpinned by evidence.

These quality standards were to be delivered through clinical governance. Professional self-regulation and lifelong learning would be encouraged. The Commission for Health Improvement (CHI) would monitor and assess the performance of the new NHS (Department of Health 1998). The government set targets to reduce mortality rates by 2010:

o—π *Keywords*

Health inequality

Health inequality exists
between social classes,
between different areas of
the country, between men
and women, and between
people from different ethnic
groups. The picture of
health inequality is clear: the
poorer you are, the more
likely you are to fall ill and
to die younger. That is the
case for almost every health
problem

o—π *Keywords*

Social class

The National Statistics
Socio-economic
Classifications is the
new occupational scale
to replace the Registrar
General's scale that
originally categorised social
class from I to V

mortality rates from cancer were to fall by one-fifth, coronary disease and stroke by two-fifths, accidents by one-fifth and suicide by one-fifth. Since then the government has added a target to halt the rise in obesity among children by 2010 (Department of Health 2004a; King's Fund 2006).

Health inequalities

Poverty and socio-economic class have been linked to **health inequalities** for many years. Edwin Chadwick showed that in 1842 the average age at death in Liverpool was 35 for landed gentry and professionals but only 15 for labourers, mechanics and servants. Although life expectancy has improved for all classes in Britain, inequalities still remain.

The Black Report, published in 1980, demonstrated that there had been continued improvement in health across all the **social classes**, but that there was still a correlation between social class, infant mortality rates and life expectancy. The death rate at most ages is two to three times higher in the lowest socio-economic group than in the highest and ill health is much greater in this group. The percentage of babies with low birth weight and the associated health problems is highest in the lowest income groups. Children in social class V are five times as likely to die from an accident as those from social class I. There is a big geographical difference in mortality between south-east England and north-west England. The North and the Midlands showed a higher rate of chronic illness than the South-east. The report acknowledged that inequalities could not be tackled by health care alone; social factors such as unemployment, poverty and housing were all important areas which needed to be considered.

Evidence base

A report from the Joseph Rowntree Foundation provides a very interesting analysis of poverty and wealth across Britain from 1968 to 2005. Go to the Foundation's website and download the findings.

The New Labour government commissioned Sir Donald Acheson to report on the inequalities in health in Britain. Published in 1998, the Acheson Report has been instrumental in fostering widespread recognition that health inequalities exist; it has been a key influence on public health policy to date. Many of the findings endorsed the 1980 Black Report and related to the differences in mortality rates between the social classes (Figures 1.3 and 1.4). However, a most significant finding indicated that the gap between the classes had in fact widened in the interim years. For example, the mortality rate among men of working age in 1970 was almost twice as high for those in class V as for those in class I. By 1990 it was three times higher and although the overall rate

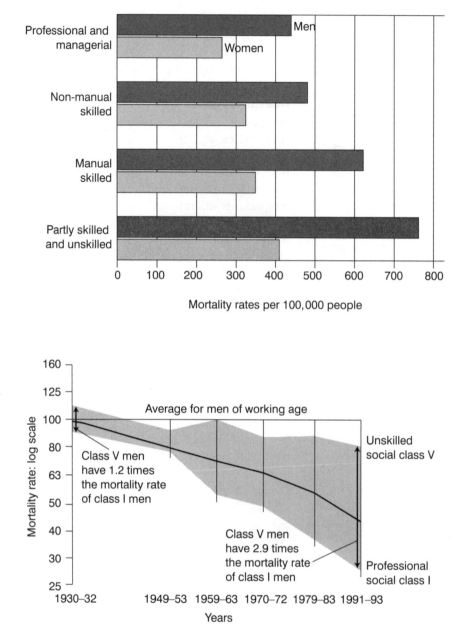

Figure 1.3 Class and mortality rates. Reprinted, with permission, from Acheson (1998)

Figure 1.4 There is a widening mortality gap between the social classes. The mortality rates are numbers of deaths per 1,000 individuals per year. Note that 1979–83 excludes 1981. Reprinted, with permission, from Department of Health (1999a)

Over to you

Obtain the Acheson Report from the Department of Health's website. Choose an area that interests you. Compare the findings in the report with the current situation and think about how, if at all, the health of the people around you has improved.

fell, it fell more among people in class I than in class V. The statistics are shocking and represent an enormous cost in human life, wasted talent and untapped potential.

The report went on to highlight a range of areas where health inequalities could be reduced. Acheson made 39 recommendations in total (of which only 3 related to the NHS) and selected 12 areas for policy development, e.g. poverty, income, employment, housing, education, young people, older people, ethnicity, and equity of services. He also recommended that all policies which influence health should be evaluated, a higher priority should be given to the health of families with children, and steps should be taken to reduce income inequalities and improve the living standard of poor households.

Saving Lives

The Acheson Report provided the context for the public health strategy in England: *Saving Lives: Our Healthier Nation* (Department of Health 1999a). The strategy aimed to prevent up to 300,000 unnecessary deaths by 2010. This was an important landmark for public health because it was the government's first public health White Paper that acknowledged the widening gap in health inequality. It emphasised a three-way partnership between individuals, communities and the state and set out an action plan to improve the health of everyone, increasing length and quality of life, and to improve the health of the worst off in society and to narrow the health gap.

The strategy was widely welcomed, although some critics felt it was still too firmly attached to a medical model of health care as it focused on four main targets based on disease: heart disease and stroke, accidents, cancer, and mental health. However, it firmly acknowledged the link between health and poverty, socio-economic circumstances and unemployment, social exclusion, lifestyle (diet, physical activities, smoking, alcohol), environmental factors (air, water, housing) and services (transport, social services, education, NHS).

It was followed by the launch of a vast number of initiatives, including health action zones, healthy living centres, Sure Start and New Deal for Communities as well as health improvement programmes. Many of the initiatives were focused on low-income families and deprived areas. It was recognised that the most effective time to intervene is in early life and that it is most effective to target areas of disadvantage and deprivation. The Sure Start initiative (Department of Health 1999a) in particular was set up to improve the health and well-being of pre-school children in deprived areas. Its targets are to halve child poverty by 2010 and to eliminate it by 2020.

It was designed to give the best start in life for every child by bringing together early education, childcare, health and family support to tackle child poverty and social exclusion, and to improve the health and well-being of families and children through local programmes to improve services for families with children under 4 and spread good practice. At the time there could be no doubt that the government was serious about tackling inequalities in health. But the plethora of initiatives and programmes, each judged on its own criteria and with separate funding, led to increasing fragmentation of services.

NHS Plan 2000

The NHS Plan (Department of Health 2000) set out the specific targets for improvement and equality of service provision. It was a modernisation plan setting out NHS strategies for the next 10 years. A small part of the plan was devoted to improving health and reducing inequalities. The priority was to focus on the root causes of poor health and inequity; partnership, cross-agency and joined-up working between government departments were seen as important. It set out plans to introduce intermediate care, modern matrons to coordinate care, better partnership working between health and social care, and the development of the patient advocacy and liaison services.

The NHS Plan emphasised the role of National Service Frameworks (NSFs) as a key driver in delivering the modernisation agenda. NSFs are designed to tackle major health issues to improve health. Each NSF is developed with the assistance of an external reference group, including health professionals, service users and carers, health service managers, partner agencies and other advocates. An NSF is designed to set national standards and identify key interventions for a defined service area or group. They put in place strategies to support the implementation of the NHS Plan and established performance milestones against which progress can be measured within an agreed timescale. Currently there are eight NSFs: mental health, coronary heart disease, cancer, older people, diabetes, children, renal care and long-term conditions. The government is consulting on a national strategy for chronic obstructive pulmonary disease (COPD) and for stroke (Department of Health 2007).

Over to you

Go to the Department of Health's website and search for the NSF that relates to your area of work. Then think about the service you provide. How does it compare to the standards set in the NSF? What are the public health implications?

Although the NHS Plan was very detailed, it made clear that yet again the government's attention was on organisational reform of the NHS. In 2001 the House of Commons Health Committee was critical of the imbalance in government policy in favour of health care as opposed to promoting health. A sense of despondency descended on the public health community when the committee acknowledged that a great opportunity to drive public health forward had been lost. According to some, public health had 'gone off the boil' (Hunter 2003, p.19).

The national health inequalities targets were finally published in 2001 and a number of priority areas were identified:

- ensuring a healthy start in life for children
- improving opportunities for children and young people
- tackling the major killer diseases – coronary heart disease and cancer
- strengthening disadvantaged communities
- addressing the wider determinants of health
- improving NHS primary care services.

Reflective activity

Think about the work you do. How does your work tackle one of the priority areas set by the government?

This was closely followed by *Tackling Health Inequalities: A Programme for Action* (Department of Health 2003), which set out a plan to reduce inequalities in health outcomes by 10 per cent as measured by infant mortality and life expectancy and to do it by 2010. Two objectives were set:

- Reduce by at least 10 per cent the gap in mortality rates for children under 1 between manual groups and the population as a whole.
- Reduce by at least 10 per cent the gap between the areas with lowest life expectancy at birth and the population as a whole.

Wanless Report

The Wanless Report, *Securing Good Health for the Whole Population*, was released in 2004 and signalled a period of significant investment and policy development for public health. Wanless focused on the prevention of ill health, tackling wider determinants of health, and the cost-effectiveness of action that can be taken to improve the health of the population, as well as reducing health inequalities. This report re-emphasises and shifts health care from acute problems to a more effective control of chronic conditions to promote maintenance of good health (Department of Health 2004a).

People are ultimately responsible for their own health and their children's health but they need to be supported to make informed decisions about their health. Wanless (2002) suggested a 'fully engaged scenario' where people consciously protect and promote their health and manage their own care. It requires a collective effort from health and care services, media, business, society, families plus the voluntary and community sector.

Public health interventions and health promotion need to be proven to be cost effective and have a solid evidence base. Clear objectives for interventions need to be set and activities should be planned. The concepts of self-care, expert patient, user involvement, community matron and community pharmacist need to be developed further to provide effective management of chronic conditions. The health service will focus on the development of primary care where health promotion and disease prevention is growing and social care is also developing to minimise the demand for health care. *The NHS Improvement Plan* (Department of Health 2004c) reaffirmed the findings of the Wanless Report and laid out a process of reform for the next 10 years and a vision for public health in 2008.

> ## Over to you
>
> Chapter 4 of *The NHS Improvement Plan* is entitled 'A Healthier and Fitter Population'. Read this chapter then say to what extent you recognise the government's vision of public health in 2008 set out on page 49.

Choosing Health

Interventions to tackle public health issues need to be more efficient to address the increase in obesity-related health issues, the slow decline in smoking rates, the growing problem of alcohol, teenage pregnancies and sexually transmitted disease, plus cancer and coronary disease. People need to be better informed to make healthier choices to improve their health. Helping people to make healthier choices is the government's new approach to public health. *Choosing Health* (Department of Health 2004a) follows the themes in the Wanless Report (Wanless 2002, 2004) on tackling public health issues. Strategies such as improving school services will support children and young people. Community matrons will help people to manage long-term conditions. A detailed delivery plan published in 2005 sets out the action plan to help children and young people to lead healthy lives and to promote healthy and active life among older people (Department of Health 2005).

This new approach has three core principles: informed choice, personalised services which are flexible and sensitive, and working together with relevant agencies, including local government, the NHS, voluntary agencies, community groups, the media and faith organisations as well as business and industries such as food, alcohol and the tobacco industry. It focuses on these priorities for action:

- reducing the numbers of people who smoke
- reducing obesity and improving diet and nutrition

- increasing exercise
- encouraging and supporting sensible drinking
- improving sexual health
- improving mental health.

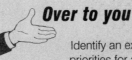

Over to you

Identify an example of a health promotion initiative for each of the six priorities for action listed immediately above.

Our Health, Our Care, Our Say

The government's focus on customer/user choice and prevention is clear in *Our Health, Our Care, Our Say* (Department of Health 2006a). Independence, choice and control are important elements in the new approach to care. However, there were some fears that focusing on personal choice may deflect attention from the importance of wider socio-economic and environmental factors that influence health, which is a recurring theme. *Our Health, Our Care, Our Say* reinforced the government's commitment to modernise social care, emphasising illness prevention and delivery of integrated health and social care (Department of Health 2006a). It provides an opportunity for community-focused, patient-led care where good health and social care are provided in the communities where people live. It promotes a better-integrated NHS and social care workforce around the needs of people who use services and supported by the common education frameworks, information systems and career frameworks in order to deliver more personalised care more effectively. Workforce issues will be fully integrated in service improvement planning by the Care Services Improvement Partnership (CSIP) and the NHS Integrated Service Improvement Programme (ISIP) (Department of Health 2006b). Here are its aims:

- Provide better prevention and early intervention for improved health, independence and well-being.
- Provide more choice and a stronger voice for individuals and communities.
- Tackle inequalities and improve access to services.
- Support people with long-term needs.

The ideas for policy development are grouped into six themes (King's Fund 2006):

- more services in the community – a local development plan will be drawn up by the local primary care trusts (PCTs) to improve services for their local people
- greater prevention

- enhanced access to general practice and community services, e.g. those with mental health issues
- better support for people with long-term conditions, integrated health and social care
- staff will be better trained with appropriate skills to provide for the ongoing needs of these clients
- provide people with a louder voice to communicate their needs.

Evidence base

Read the summary of *Our Health, Our Care, Our Say*.

The next decade

As the NHS approaches its sixtieth anniversary in July 2008, the prime minister has announced an unprecedented review to establish a vision for the next decade of the health service. At the heart of the review is a service that will be based less on central direction and more on patient and service user control, choice and local accountability. It is envisaged that this will ensure services are responsive to the public and local communities (Department of Health 2007). Another range of policies is surely on the way.

Key points   Top tips

- The environmental change era, 1850–1900, emphasised improving sanitation and working conditions
- The personal preventive era, 1900–1930, emphasised maternal and child welfare
- The therapeutic era, 1930–1970, developed medical interventions and illness services
- The new public health era, from 1970 onwards, acknowledged the need to tackle inequalities in health and broader health-harming issues

How policy affects practitioners

It is not easy to see a clear pattern in how the health-care professional's role is developing to keep pace with the development of public health. There has been almost a blizzard of initiatives since 1997, and as health gain is measured in the long term, it is difficult to say what has and has not worked. Measuring health gains and health outcomes can be difficult, time consuming and resource demanding. Our own understanding of nursing is changing and responding to changes in society, policy development and service direction. All of this happens at a time when there is a need to tackle longer-term and preventive issues within a policy context that is often driven by shorter-term pressures.

There are societal pressures that make it difficult for long-term issues to be addressed in full. The cycle between elections is five years at most. Governments often look for short-term solutions to demonstrate success. The mass media can have a huge impact on health choices made by the public. Over 80 per cent of the population cited the media as their most important source of health information (Office of Health Economics 1994). However, pressure from mass media can also direct policy makers to focus on the visible and dramatic agendas such as long waiting lists and hospital bed shortages, rather than putting resources and effort into promoting health. And in a system where failure is exposed relentlessly, there can be an unwillingness to experiment with new approaches or to take risks.

In nursing and other areas of health care, an understanding of public health and public health policies provides a structure, direction and drive for improving health. Promoting health not only helps to prevent illness, but can also reduce hospital admissions, which shortens hospital waiting lists, and hospital waiting lists are a prime driver in the current NHS modernisation. There is a misconception that public health and health promotion belong solely to those who work in primary health care. There is a need to develop a stronger focus of public health in all nursing and health-care practice. This theme is developed in Chapters 2 and 3, which look in detail at the principles of public health practice and public health approaches to nursing.

Conclusion

This chapter briefly examined the origins and development of public health. It gave details of policy development in the past 50 years, particularly the policy context of the government over the past 10 years (Table 1.1 overleaf). The social, economic and environmental influence on health emerged as a dominant theme throughout history. Successive governments have attempted to address these issues through health and social policies. The present government recognises and accepts the link between poverty and health and has introduced policy initiatives that try to reduce inequalities in health.

Improving health is a long-term commitment that requires long-term strategies. All nurses and health-care professionals have a role to play in improving the public's health. Boundaries are blurred between primary and secondary care delivery and between health and social care. Integration of care delivery emphasises the importance of collaborative practice of all health and social care staff within and between primary and secondary care as well as with other government departments and voluntary sectors. These boundaries are further blurred when one considers the wider activities – housing, transport, leisure, environment – that underpin a wider, more holistic definition of health.

Table 1.1 Key public health policies 1997–2007

Year	Report or announcement	Action
1997	*The New NHS: Modern, Dependable*	A Labour government appoints a public health minister. Commitment to tackling inequalities in health
1998	Acheson Report	Confirmed the findings of the Black Report and found that the gap had widened since the Black Report's publication in 1980
1999	*Saving Lives: Our Healthier Nation*	National strategy for public health. Four target areas: circulatory disease and stroke, accidents, cancer, mental health
2000	*The NHS Plan*	Further organisational change in the NHS created national service frameworks, primary care groups and health improvement programmes
2003	*Tackling Health Inequalities*	Plan to reduce inequalities in health outcomes by 10% as measured by infant mortality and life expectancy at birth
2004	Wanless Report	Identified the 'fully engaged' scenario as the way to ensure action on inequalities in health
2004	NHS Plan for Improvement	Public health vision for 2008 and a healthier and fitter population
2004	*Choosing Health*	Six targets: improve nutrition and reduce obesity, reduce accidents, reduce smoking, reduce drinking, mental health, sexual health
2006	*Our Health, Our Care, Our Say*	Aim to give patients and service users more control over the treatment they receive – choice and voice
2007	Prime minister announces a comprehensive review of the NHS	Establish a vision for the next 10 years

Health care is not just about treating illnesses, but is also about promoting positive health to prevent illness. Practitioners in different disciplines need to look at their public health role and develop new ways of working to incorporate the understanding of public health and health promotion strategies within the health-care services they deliver.

ꓡꓡꓡꓡ*Rapid recap*

Check your progress so far by working through each of the following questions.

1. What are the five common causes of death in recent years?
2. What are the four main eras of public health development?
3. What are the four target areas in the White Paper *Saving Lives*?
4. What are the six target areas in the White Paper *Choosing Health*?

If you have difficulty understanding more than one of the questions, read through the section again to refresh your understanding before moving on.

References

Acheson, D. (1988) *Public Health in England: The Report of the Committee of Inquiry into the Future Development of the Public Health Function.* HMSO, London.

Acheson, D. (1998) *Independent Inquiry into Inequality in Health: Report.* HMSO, London.

Baggott, R. (2000) *Public Health: Policy and Politics.* Macmillan, Basingstoke, Hants.

Black, D., Morris, J., Smith, C. and Townsend, P. (1980) *Inequalities in Health: Report of a Working Party.* Department of Health and Social Security, London.

Chadwick, E. (1842) Report on the Sanitary Condition of the Labouring Population of Great Britain. Poor Law Commission, London. Cited in Baggott, R. (2000) *Public Health, Policy and Politics.* Macmillan, Basingstoke, Hants.

Department of Health (1992) *The Health of the Nation: A Strategy for Health.* HMSO, London.

Department of Health (1997) *The New NHS: Modern, Dependable.* HMSO, London.

Department of Health (1998) *A First-Class Service: Quality in the New NHS.* HMSO, London.

Department of Health (1999a) *Saving Lives: Our Healthier Nation.* HMSO, London.

Department of Health (1999b) *National Service Framework for Mental Health.* HMSO, London.

Department of Health (2000) *The NHS Plan.* HMSO, London.

Department of Health (2001a) *National Service Framework for Diabetes.* HMSO, London.

Department of Health (2001b) *The Expert Patient: A New Approach to Chronic Disease Management for the 21st Century.* HMSO, London.

Department of Health (2001c) *National Service Framework for Older People.* HMSO, London.

Department of Health (2003) *Tackling Health Inequalities: A Programme for Action.* HMSO, London.

Department of Health (2004a) *Choosing Health: Making Healthier Choices Easier.* HMSO, London.

Department of Health (2004b) *National Service Framework for Children.* HMSO, London.

Department of Health (2004c) *The NHS Improvement Plan: Putting People at the Heart of Public Services.* HMSO, London.

Department of Health (2005) *National Service Framework for Long-Term Conditions.* HMSO, London.

Department of Health (2006a) *Our Health, Our Care, Our Say.* HMSO, London.

Department of Health (2006b) *Integrated Service Improvement Plans: Realising Quality and Value for Money.* HMSO, London.

Department of Health (2007) Shaping health care for the next decade. Press release on www.gnn.gov.uk, accessed 10 July 2007.

Ham, C. (2004) *Health Policy in Britain*, 5th edn. Palgrave Macmillan, Basingstoke, Hants.

Health Development Agency (2004) *Health Needs Assesment.* HDA, London.

Holland, W. and Stewart, S. (1998) *Public Health: The Vision and the Challenge.* Nuffield Trust, London.

Hunter, D. J. (1999) Public health policies. In: *Perspectives in Public Health* (eds Griffiths, S. and Hunter, D. J.). Radcliffe, Oxford.

Hunter, D. J. (2003) *Public Health Policy.* Blackwell Publishing, Oxford.

King's Fund (2006) Public health briefing on *Our Health, Our Care, Our Say.*

Klein, R. (1980) Between nihilism and utopia in health care. Unpublished lecture, Yale University.

Koelen, M. and Van den Ban, A. (2004) *Health Education and Health Promotion*. Wageningen Academic, Wageningen.

Lalonde, M. (1974) *A New Perspective on the Health of Canadians*. Ministry of National Health and Welfare, Ottawa.

Office for National Statistics (2006) *Most Common Cause of Death*. ONS, London.

Office of Health Economics (1994) *Health and the Consumer*. OHE, London.

Orme, J., Powell, J., Taylor, P., Harrison, T. and Grey, M. (2003) *Public Health for the 21st Century*. Open University Press, Maidenhead, Berks.

Rosen, G. (1993) *A History of Public Health*. Johns Hopkins, Baltimore MD.

Shaw, M. (1994) *Global Society and International Relations*. Polity Press, Cambridge.

Smith, A. and Jacobson, B. (1988) *The Nation's Health: A Strategy for the 1990s*. King Edward's Hospital Fund, London.

Tang, K. C., Beaglehole, R. and Leeuw, E. (2006) Sixth Global Conference on Health Promotion, Bangkok, August 2005. *Health Promotion International,* **21**, Supplement 1, December 2006.

United Nations (1993) *Agenda 21: Earth Summit – The United Nations Programme of Action from Rio*. United Nations Publication.

Wanless, D. (2002) *Securing Our Future Health*. HM Treasury, London.

Wanless, D. (2004) *Securing Good Health for the Whole Population*. HMSO, London.

World Health Organization (1984) *Health Promotion: A Discussion Document on the Concepts and Principles.* WHO, Copenhagen.

World Health Organization (1986) *Ottawa Charter for Health Promotion*. WHO, Geneva.

World Health Organization (1988) *Second International Conference on Health Promotion, Adelaide: Recommendations*. WHO/Australian Department of Community Services and Health, Adelaide.

World Health Organization (1991) *Third International Conference on Health Promotion: Sundsvall Statement on Supportive Environment for Health*. WHO/UNEP/Nordic Council of Ministers, Sundsvall.

World Health Organization (1997) *The Jakarta Declaration on Leading Health Promotion into the 21st Century*. WHO, Geneva.

World Health Organization (2000) *Report on the Fifth Global Conference on Health Promotion Bridging the Equity Gap. 5–9th June 2000*, Mexico City. WHO, Geneva.

2
Principles and key concepts in public health practice

Ann Day

Learning outcomes

By the end of this chapter you should be able to:

★ Understand the different concepts associated with public health

★ Describe the key principles of public health practice

★ Relate the principles of public health practice to individual, family, group, community and population concepts of public health

★ Identify the multidimensional influences on health and well-being.

Introduction

Chapter 1 showed that since New Labour came to power in 1997, public health has been high on the government's agenda (Acheson 1998; Department of Health 1997, 1999a, 1999b, 2000, 2004, 2006; Home Office 1998; Wanless 2002, 2004). Simultaneously, public health practice particularly in nursing, has gained recognition and enhanced credibility (Acheson 1998; Department of Health 1999b, 2001a, 2004, 2006; Home Office 1998). Some people might think that public health is a relatively new area of nursing practice, but nurses have always made a contribution to public health, especially nurses working in the community (Carr and Davidson 2004; Standing Nursing and Midwifery Advisory Committee 1995). Indeed the first public health nurses were the ladies sanitary inspectors, who in 1867 were working with disadvantaged mothers and their children in the slums of Salford. Over the past 140 years these practitioners have transmogrified into what we now call specialist community public health nurses (SCPHNs) (Nursing and Midwifery Council 2004). While SCPHNs remain key public health practitioners working with individuals, families and communities to tackle health inequalities, they are now part of a much wider, multidisciplinary public health practitioner workforce (Department of Health 2001b) as follows:

- **public health specialists** – a small group of people from a variety of professional backgrounds and experience, such as consultant public health nurses.

- **public health practitioners** – spend a substantial part of their time furthering health by directly working with groups and communities (examples are health visitors, school health advisers, occupational health nurses, environmental health officers, community development workers).
- **public health wider (non-specialist) workers** – including managers in the NHS and local authorities, nurses, midwives, teachers and other health workers such as health trainers.

With public health now firmly on the government agenda, all nurses are encouraged to become more involved in public health, whatever their clinical practice. Whether nursing on a neonatal unit or nursing on an older people's unit, public health is everybody's business. Public health has adapted its practice over the years to embrace contemporary public health approaches and works in collaboration with populations, but more fundamentally with the individuals, families and communities who make up those populations. The main focus of public health practice is very much concerned with improving the health of populations, preventing disease, promoting health and reducing inequalities.

The principles of public health practice

Biomedical model and social model

To understand the principles of public health practice, we need to consider the key concepts in public health and more fully understand Acheson's definition of public health: 'the science and art of preventing disease, prolonging life, promoting, protecting and improving health and well-being through the organised efforts of society' (Acheson 1988, p.16).

The definition of public health highlights several key concepts fundamental to public health, which will be unpacked and outlined. Firstly, the 'science' or biomedical model and the 'art' or social model approaches to health. While these models can be seen as two distinct models, public health nursing simultaneously takes account of both approaches. To understand the health of a community, it is essential to understand the data on mortality (death) and morbidity (ill health) for that community, which is the epidemiology of disease. **Health needs assessments** are conducted by public health practitioners to identify and assess health conditions and the health needs of a community. Here are some of the questions explored in a health needs assessment:

- How many people are in the community?
- How many are affected by a specific disease such as coronary heart disease?
- What are the ages of those affected?

⌐⊶ᴛ Keywords

Health needs assessment

A health needs assessment is a systematic approach to determine the health issues facing a population, leading to an agreed service or intervention which is intended to improve health and reduce inequalities (Health Development Agency 2004)

- Are men and women equally affected?
- Is there a common pattern?

The data from the health needs assessment is then analysed to determine the occurrence of coronary heart disease and the effective, evidence-based interventions that should be made available to the community.

Besides this biomedical model, sometimes known as the epidemiological model, it is also important to consider the social model to fully grasp what is affecting the health and well-being of the community. For example, is there an inequality? In other words, is there a gap between the most advantaged sections of society and the least advantaged? Here are some specific questions to ask for the coronary heart disease example:

- Is there an inequality in those presenting with coronary heart disease?
- Do they live in a disadvantaged area?
- Is unemployment high?
- Is there poor accessibility to shops selling good, healthy food at reasonable prices?
- Is there good accessibility to health-care services?

A key principle of public health from a nursing perspective is to practise within an overarching framework which links the two models to give an overall picture of the health and well-being of the individuals and the whole community.

Reflective activity

Think about patients with coronary heart disease that you have nursed or cared for in some other way. Is there any commonality between them? Here are some questions you could ask:

- If they have a job, is it a skilled or unskilled job?
- What are the shops like in the neighbourhood where they live?
- Is there a nearby park or open space where people can walk without feeling afraid?

Health protection and promotion

If we think of the biomedical model and the social model of public health as an overarching framework for understanding public health practice, we can then start to think about the main principles of public health in the second part of Acheson's definition: 'preventing disease, prolonging life, promoting, protecting ... health'. These key public health principles translate into the three strands of health protection, health promotion and the maintenance or restoration of health.

Building on the example of coronary heart disease, here are some things that the public health practitioner might be involved in:

- **health protection** – working with the local community and the local authority to dissuade local shopkeepers from selling cigarettes or alcohol to under-age children
- **health promotion** – in collaboration with the local community, setting up sessions to help and support people wanting to change to a healthier lifestyle, such as stopping smoking or losing weight
- **maintaining or restoring health** – provision of screening programmes, such as blood pressure sessions, in the local community centre, the local shopping centre or other accessible places.

Wanless (2004) warned that it might be difficult to encourage some sections of society, particularly disadvantaged groups, to become 'fully engaged' with some of these activities. As a result, the government (Department of Health 2004) suggested that the delivery must be underpinned by three principles:

- **Informed choice for all** – people need to have good, reliable information so they can make choices that affect their health.
- **Personalisation of support to make healthy choices** – public health practitioners must consider the reality of people's lives when giving help and support. It makes no sense to encourage someone to go running when that person doesn't feel safe to be out and about in their local neighbourhood.
- **Partnership working to make health everybody's business** – this includes working not only in partnership with individuals and communities but also with the public, the private and voluntary sectors, the media and many other groups.

Over to you

Go to the Health Protection Agency website and see which areas of your practice have a health protection element.

Health and well-being of people and communities

The phrase 'improving health and well-being' is another key public health concept and fundamental to public health practice. The idea is as old as civilisation itself. The Romans focused on the health and well-being of their populations, with sophisticated, safe water supplies and latrines back in 3000 BC. Aristotle in 384 BC used the Greek word *eudamonia*, 'the well-being of the whole person'. Twenty-four centuries later, public health policy and public health practice encompass not only the well-being of the whole person as an individual, but also that person's family, the community where they live and the population or society they belong to.

In public health terms, 'well-being' means being concerned with people's health within a holistic interpretation of health; that is, incorporating the physical, mental, emotional and social aspects of health. This well-being of the individual cannot be seen in isolation, but is interconnected with and interdependent on their family, community, population and the policies and systems that operate not only at a national level, but also at a local level. These seemingly disparate yet connected areas can have beneficial or harmful effects on a person's health and well-being.

Case study

Oliver twist

Read this extract from the *Guardian* (18 September 2006) then answer the questions.

Parents and head in school dinner talks

Two mothers who handed out fast food to school children in a backlash against a school's healthy eating policy will meet the school's headteacher today in [an] attempt to resolve the row.

Julie Critchlow and Sam Walker have been accused of undermining the Jamie Oliver inspired crusade against junk food in schools by handing out burgers, fish and chips, and fizzy drinks through the fence at Rawmarsh Comprehensive School, in Rotherham, South Yorkshire.

They say they are giving children what they want after the school brought in a new healthy menu and banned pupils from going to local takeaways.

But they also insist that they favour healthy eating, pointing out that they have also handed out jacket potatoes and salad sandwiches.

- What are your thoughts on what the two mothers did?
- What do you think about the school bringing in a new healthy menu?
- What might be the long-term holistic outcomes for the children's health and well-being?

Collaboration and partnership

The final part of Acheson's definition, 'through the organised efforts of society', refers to collaborative working with communities and multidisciplinary agencies to achieve better health and well-being. The idea is that the community itself needs to participate actively in determining the main issues affecting its health and well-being. This means that the community and people in the community need to feel empowered and confident enough to articulate their issues. This can often be a problem in disadvantaged areas where some people may feel that they have no control over their lives and can do nothing to affect what happens to them. This is known as an external locus of control (Rotter 1966). A locus of control is the extent to which individuals believe they can control events that affect them. People who have an internal locus of control believe that they have some control over their lives and therefore have some self-confidence and self-esteem. An important principle of public health practice is to work closely with people and communities, helping to build up their confidence so they can take an active role in decision-making processes that affect their community and work effectively with professionals.

However, a community's ideas about what it needs might differ from the professional agencies' ideas about what it needs. For example, a community might think that their biggest problem is concern about drug misuse or crime in the area, and the related concern about letting their children move about freely. But the agencies – health agencies, local authorities, voluntary organisations and latterly the private sector – may be influenced by the government agenda focusing on obesity as a major public health problem. The key to collaborative working and partnerships is to reach a common understanding of what might be the priorities and how best to tackle them. Chapter 7 discusses partnership working in more detail.

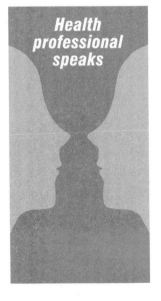

Health professional speaks

Health visitor

As a local community development worker and a health visitor, I had been given a remit based on the government's Respect Agenda to set up a parenting programme to try and prevent children becoming the 'juvenile delinquents' of the future. But when I asked the mothers what they wanted, they said they wanted to feel good – they wanted to be pampered. So I used part of the funding to set up some aromatherapy, beauty and manicure sessions. Every mother who came along could choose three sessions of whatever she wanted. In time the group became quite a close-knit group and continued to meet, even though the funding for feel-good sessions had run out. They started to share among themselves the problems they'd been having as parents. We heard each other's stories and discussed things that we found had worked and things that hadn't worked, and in our own we way developed a parenting programme based on the mothers' strategies to cope with difficult parenting situations.

A new 'citizen' model of involvement has been devised which encourages active involvement and gives a 'voice' as well as 'choice' (Department of Health 2006) and ownership of services for the community. Known as 'social enterprise', the model is based on members of the community influencing the planning, design and delivery of health-care services and also being part-owners alongside patients, staff and other organisations, including private and commercial organisations.

Evidence base

For further information on community empowerment, read Graney, A. (2002) Effectiveness and community empowerment. In: *Public Health in Policy and Practice* (ed. Cowley, S.). Ballière Tindall, London.
To read more on social enterprise go to the King's Fund website and read the working paper 'Social enterprise and community-based care' by Richard Lewis, Peter Hunt and David Carson.
Also go to the Department of Health website and search for 'social enterprise'.

Working with inequalities

A key concept of public health practice is working with individuals and communities to reduce inequalities in health. Wanless (2004) issued this warning:

> Persistent socio-economic inequalities in the UK, combined with a greater severity of market failures affecting lower socio-economic groups, seem to have contributed to significant inequalities in health outcomes which, unless tackled, will present a significant barrier to many in society becoming 'fully engaged'.

Health experiences differ between different social and economic groups, geographical areas, genders, cultures and ethnic communities. These inequalities in health in the UK are widening, despite a general improvement in the health of the nation over the past 30 years. The stark reality of this means that in 1997–1999 the life expectancy at birth for a man in a professional occupation was 7.4 years higher than for a man in an unskilled manual occupation (Office for National Statistics 2005). Similarly, in 1999–2001 Glasgow City was the local authority with the lowest life expectancy at birth for both males and females. Male life expectancy was 68.7, 10 years less than for North Dorset local authority at 79.3.

A thorough understanding of the causes of these inequalities is vital for anyone who wishes to work in the field of public health. Dahlgren and Whitehead (1991) explored the interaction of complex, multidimensional influences that affect people's health. They produced a now famous 'rainbow' model which highlights the main determinants of health and helps us understand how inequalities occur (Figure 2.1).

Age, sex and constitutional factors

When Dahlgren and Whitehead produced their rainbow model, it was thought that the factors at the centre of the model were fixed characteristics and could not be changed. However, with the tremendous advances in genetic technology, this situation may be changing. A person in the centre is born at a certain time, either male or female, of a

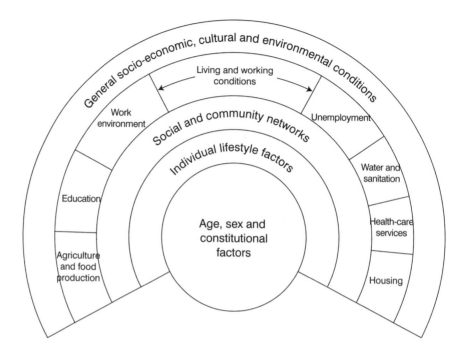

Figure 2.1 Determinants of health. Reprinted, with permission, from Dahlgren and Whitehead (1991)

Within the figure:

General socio-economic, cultural and environmental conditions

Living and working conditions

Social and community networks

Individual lifestyle factors

Work environment

Unemployment

Education

Water and sanitation

Health-care services

Agriculture and food production

Housing

Age, sex and constitutional factors

particular ethnic group and may have inherited genetic factors that may affect aspects of their health and development. Also, they may have been subject to smoking, alcohol or drug misuse in utero.

Individual lifestyle factors

In the next layer of the model, the choices the person makes about their lifestyle as they grow into adulthood can have a positive or negative effect on their health. For example, if they drink heavily, smoke, eat unhealthy foods and take little or no exercise, they will be affecting their health in a detrimental way and they will be predisposed to coronary heart disease.

Social and community networks

Within current government policy, this layer of the rainbow model is seen as vitally important for the health and well-being of a person, their family and their community. Having friends, relatives, friendly neighbours and feeling safe in the community are thought to provide people with a sense of belonging and a feeling that a supportive network is close at hand. This social capital encourages trust and reciprocity in the community; it is a key public health concept (page 31). Public health practitioners can work with local communities to support them in determining their community needs; for example, the community could decide that a priority is to find a place where children can play safely.

Living and working conditions

The living and working conditions layer of the rainbow model relates to some of the most important influences on the health of individuals and communities; it focuses on the local economy and the conditions in which people live and work. Many issues may be beyond the control of individuals and communities and some may influence their health in a detrimental way. For example, communities may live in food deserts, where it is difficult to buy good, healthy food at reasonable prices. Poor public transport links may affect access to good food, jobs, education, health services and social care. It is a sad irony that disadvantaged people often do not access health and care services, although they would actually benefit more than the worried well, who make frequent access. This inverse care law (Tudor-Hart 1971) is not just about physical accessibility, but also about the availability of good health and social care services plus the welcome given to disadvantaged people when they do access these services.

Moreover, an area may have poor educational facilities. Poor educational facilities seldom attract better teachers and this may affect the educational attainment of children. Education and skills are thought to be essential for escaping a lifetime of disadvantage. The fundamental ethos underpinning the government's Sure Start programme is that an early start to education, together with childcare, health and family support services, encourages a child's learning and will help them avoid a life of disadvantage. Housing may be poor, damp and without basic heating. Unemployment may be a key issue, with the closure of local factories that employed the community. Or a person may be in low-paid employment with poor conditions. Separately or combined, all these factors can affect people's physical, mental and emotional health.

Health professional speaks

Health visitor

I am an experienced health visitor and I used to run a free parents and tots session at the local community hall. I was very upset when I found out that the local council wanted to close the hall. Over the five years when I ran the sessions, I noticed there was much less post-natal depression and generally fewer mental health problems. The local council said it had to close the hall as it was 'unsafe' but there was going to be a 'bigger and much smarter' building where it would put together health, social care and education professionals. The planners put it three kilometres from the old community hall and there was no regular bus service. It was not on the way to the local shops, schools or any other amenities. The parents and tots sessions at the new hall ceased after six months as nobody went along.

Socio-economic, cultural and environmental conditions

The final layer is for the overarching political strategies that dictate policy, economic and environmental issues and that partly influence our views on culture, ethnicity and gender. The strategies depend on which political ideology is current. So, as explained in Chapter 1, New Labour governments have introduced a huge array of policies that focus on community involvement to improve public health in the UK.

Reflective activity

Study Figure 2.2 and think about the children growing up in this environment.

● What might be some of the risks they are susceptible to?

● What might be some of the influences within the family that the children are subjected to that might be harmful to their health and well-being?

● What sort of issues within the community might this family be struggling to cope with that could potentially affect their long-term health and well-being?

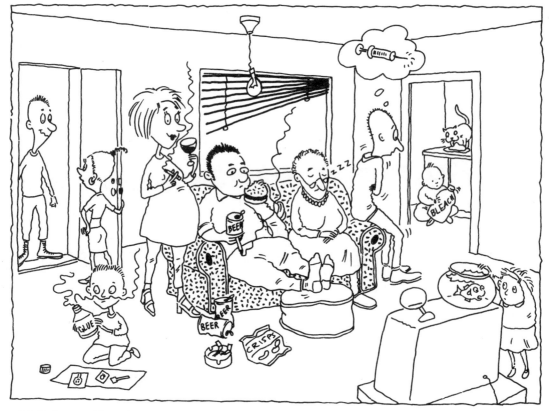

Figure 2.2 Reflect on this environment

Strengthening communities through social capital

Here is how the World Health Organization (1998) has defined social capital:

> Social capital represents the degree of social cohesion in communities. It refers to the processes between people that establish networks, norms and social trust, and facilitate(s) coordination and cooperation for mutual benefit.

Social capital is thought to encourage social cohesion and increase the likelihood of individuals and communities being socially included rather than excluded through, for example, disadvantage and unemployment. Employment is thought to be a key impetus that gives a sense of well-being, participation and a social network of friends or colleagues. As Puttnam (2003) suggests, social capital has positive economic effects and these economic effects have a knock-on effect in that a thriving local economy will encourage social capital by providing jobs.

The Health Development Agency (2004) suggested that social capital has four key elements:

- **social resources** – such as informal arrangements between neighbours or within a faith community
- **collective resources** – such as self-help groups, credit unions and community safety schemes
- **economic resources** – such as levels of employment and access to green, open spaces
- **cultural resources** – such as libraries, arts centres and local schools.

Reflective activity

Social capital is an important public health concept that is thought to have positive effects on health and well-being. Look at this quotation from Robert Puttnam (2003), the great exponent of social capital: 'We are social animals: for example there is the extraordinary statistic that if you presently do not belong to any group, joining a club or society of some kind halves the risk that you will die in the next year.'

- What do you think about this statement?
- What might be some of the challenges facing the family in the cartoon on page 30 if they wanted to join a group?

Social capital remains a challenge, particularly in some disadvantaged areas, where social exclusion is rife. Social exclusion has been described as 'what can happen when individuals or areas face a combination of linked problems such as unemployment, discrimination, poor skills, low incomes, poor housing, high crime, bad health and family breakdown' (Social Exclusion Unit 2004). Lone parents and their children are a particular group who can face social exclusion. According to the Office for National Statistics (2005), in 2003 a quarter of all children in the UK lived with one parent, and 43 per cent of those parents were not in employment.

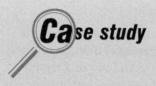

Case study

Jan and Jade

Jan, aged 18, lives in a one-bedroom council flat in a disadvantaged inner-city area with her daughter Jade, aged 2. She can't get a job as she hasn't any qualifications and she has no one who can look after Jade. Jan was at school studying for her GCSEs when she became pregnant. She'd been having a difficult time at home, not getting on with her mother, who'd taken up with Jed, 10 years younger than her mum. Jed gave Jan the creeps, especially when he suggested that he'd moved in to be closer to Jan, not her mother.

Jan started to bunk off school and hang about with a few people older than her who'd left school a couple of years before. She got pregnant. The school didn't seem very interested but Jan was given some home tuition. Jan didn't like spending too much time at home because Jed was there. She left home and ended up in a place for young mums and babies. Eventually she got a council flat. She finds it very difficult living on benefits. She wants to buy Jade things like nice clothes and healthy food but she can't afford them. Jan can buy a packet of custard cream biscuits for the same price as one apple and Jade seems much happier with custard creams. Jan knows that she shouldn't smoke, but she thinks it helps her cope with her loneliness and boredom.

- From a public health perspective, what could have been done to avoid Jan becoming socially excluded?
- What can the public health practitioner do to enable Jan and Jade to become socially included?

Keywords

Upstream

Upstream public health practice focuses on preventive measures, tackling the root causes of ill health. It brings a wide range of benefits in an attempt to improve health

Downstream

Downstream public health practice focuses on tackling existing health problems. It brings a narrower range of benefits with direct effects for the individual

Upstream and downstream health strategies

A well-known analogy considers public health strategies as either **upstream** or **downstream** on a river (Acheson 1998). Acheson talked about upstream causes of ill health such as poverty and social exclusion. Upstream strategies to combat these inequalities are policies which lead to health interventions to prevent the development of avoidable diseases and improve the health of individuals and communities. A good example is the recent smoking ban in restaurants and pubs in the UK. Meanwhile, downstream on the river, smoking, unhealthy diets and lack of exercise are all causes of ill health. Downstream strategies focus on individual lifestyle factors and interventions to treat preventable disease such as support for people to help them quit smoking and classes that teach people to cook healthy food.

Over to you

Recent public health policies (Department of Health 2004) have been criticised for laying too much emphasis on the individual's responsibility for health. Several complex factors influence our health, and we may have little influence over some factors. The UK Public Health Association (2004) produced a critical analysis of *Choosing Health*. Read this extract from the UKPHA analysis and work out your own views on the subject.

The relevance of choice in public health

We welcome the recognition given in the White Paper to the legitimate role of government in creating healthier environments and shifting social norms in order to support individuals and protect the health of vulnerable groups. However, we fundamentally disagree with the portrayal of personal choice as the key issue for improved public health and the focus within the White Paper on individuals as consumers, and not as citizens.

What does choice mean in public health? Public health is principally about organising society for the good of the population's health; at this level of concern, it is no more a matter of individual choice than the weather.

Many individuals cannot choose whether or not they have sufficient income to live in warm safe housing and eat healthy food. They cannot choose to walk or cycle when both pedestrian and cycle routes are often neither safe nor pleasant and dominated by the needs of the car. Those who suffer the worst health inequalities cannot choose to enjoy the benefits of local safe green spaces to pursue healthy outdoor activities or to breathe clean fresh air.

Even when choice can be exercised, consumer decisions are profoundly affected and influenced by the powerful and all pervasive impact of the advertising and promotional activities of the food and drink industry, which is driven by the need to increase sales and maximize shareholder value rather than to promote the public's health.

Conclusion

Public health is a key part of health provision in the twenty-first century. It is the business of every nurse and health-care practitioner, whether they work in an A & E department or a surgical unit. Public health practice is not only concerned with individual people, but also with the families and groups they belong to, the communities where they live, and the population or society they are part of. Public health's main concern is to improve the health and well-being of people by preventing disease, by promoting health and by striving to reduce inequalities. Moreover, public health practice does not happen in isolation. The ethos underpinning public health practice is one of partnership and collaboration with other agencies, but more importantly, with the individuals, groups and communities who need the public health interventions.

RRRRRapid recap

Check your progress so far by working through each of the following questions.

1. What are the main principles of public health practice?
2. What is meant by a community?
3. How might a public health practitioner gather information about the health of a community?
4. How can the area where a family lives affect the family's health?

If you have difficulty understanding more than one of the questions, read through the section again to refresh your understanding before moving on.

References

Acheson, D. (1988) *Public Health in England: The Report of the Committee of Inquiry into the Future Development of the Public Health Function.* HMSO, London.

Acheson, D. (1998) *Independent Inquiry into Inequality in Health: Report.* HMSO, London.

Carr, S. and Davidson, A. (2004) Public health nursing: developing practice. *Practice Development in Health Care,* **3**(2) 101–112.

Dahlgren, G. and Whitehead, M. (1991) *Policies and Strategies to Promote Social Equity in Health.* Institute of Future Studies, Stockholm.

Department of Health (1997) *The New NHS: Modern, Dependable.* HMSO, London.

Department of Health (1999a) *Saving Lives: Our Healthier Nation.* HMSO, London.

Department of Health (1999b) *Making a Difference: Strengthening the Nursing, Midwifery and Health Visiting Contribution to Health and Health Care.* HMSO, London.

Department of Health (2000) *The NHS Plan.* HMSO, London.

Department of Health (2001a) *Health Visitor Practice Development pack.* HMSO, London.

Department of Health (2001b) *Report of the Chief Medical Officer's Project to Strengthen the Public Health Function.* HMSO, London.

Department of Health (2004) *Choosing Health: Making Healthier Choices Easier.* HMSO, London.

Department of Health (2006) *Our Health, Our Care, Our Say.* HMSO, London.

Graney, A. (2002) Effectiveness and community empowerment. In: *Public Health in Policy and Practice* (ed. Cowley, S.). Ballière Tindall, London.

Health Development Agency (2004) *Health Needs Assessment.* HDA, London.

Home Office. (1998) *Supporting Families: A Consultation Document.* HMSO, London.

Nursing and Midwifery Council (2004) *Standards of Proficiency for Specialist Community Public Health Nurses.* NMC, London.

Office for National Statistics. (2005) Census 2001 profiles. www.statistics.gov.uk/census 2001/profiles/printV/00CH.asp, accessed 27 February 2006.

Puttnam, R. (2003) Social capital. Lecture given at the Royal Society.

Rotter, J. (1966) Generalized expectancies for internal versus external control of reinforcements. *Psychological Monographs*, **80**, no. 609.

Social Exclusion Unit (2004) *Breaking the Cycle: Taking Stock of Progress and Priorities for the Future*. Office of the Deputy Prime Minister, London.

Standing Nursing and Midwifery Advisory Committee (1995) *Making it Happen*. Department of Health, London.

Tudor-Hart, J. (1971) The inverse care law. *Lancet*, **1**, 405–412.

United Kingdom Public Health Association (2004) *Choosing Health or Losing Health?* UKPHA, London.

Wanless, D. (2002) *Securing Our Future Health*. HM Treasury, London.

Wanless, D. (2004) *Securing Good Health for the Whole Population*. HMSO, London.

World Health Organization (1998) *Health Promotion Glossary*. WHO, Geneva.

3
Public health approaches to practice

Susan M. Carr and **Ann Day**

Learning outcomes

By the end of this chapter you should be able to:

★ Identify areas in which you already contribute a public health approach to practice

★ Identify areas in which you can further develop public health in your practice

★ Describe the overlap between general nursing practice and the public health approach to practice

★ Determine how to develop a bigger contribution to public health in your practice

★ Understand the different key areas of public health practice, models and the skills of public health.

Introduction

Chapters 1 and 2 explained that public health is everybody's business. The public health workforce contains a wide spectrum of practitioners working at different levels to improve health and reduce health inequalities. Practitioners come from diverse backgrounds in health, social care, education, transport, environment, housing and agriculture, and they work in the public, voluntary and private sectors. Recent health policy documents, such as *Choosing Health* (Department of Health 2004a) and *Our Health, Our Care, Our Say* (Department of Health 2006a), endorse this message and they endorse the need for all practitioners to more fully appreciate and realise their public health role. A practitioner may still need to practise public health even if their job title does not contain the words 'public health'.

As you read this chapter, you will see how some areas of public health practice are practised by all practitioners across the three parts of the Nursing and Midwifery Council (NMC) register. Scenarios and case studies will help show you how the theory of public health can be put into practice and help you to start thinking about how much of your practice could be classified as public health practice. You may then be able to enhance your public health practice by developing different types of knowledge and skills. To help you in this process, we will explore public health approaches to practice by exposing some of the component parts: the key areas of public health practice, some public health models, and the skills to practise public health. We will discuss them individually, assemble them into a whole, then use a diagram and a case study to show how they interconnect.

Analyse current practice

Public health is about improving health in its widest holistic sense and that is why many nurses, practitioners and managers are already working this way. But busy practitioners do not always recognise the public health aspect of their practice. The spheres of practice in Figure 3.1 can help people understand their vital contribution to public health and then develop it further. Some practitioners are largely in the sphere of general nursing, such as a staff nurse in A & E; other practitioners are largely in the sphere of public health nursing, such as an occupational health nurse in a large supermarket chain. But even for these practitioners, some of their work will overlap into the other sphere. The A & E nurse will do some public health nursing and the supermarket nurse will do some general nursing.

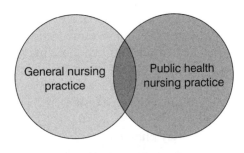

Figure 3.1 Spheres of practice

Reflective activity

To begin reflecting on your contribution to public health, start by thinking about how you practise and how the service you work in guides you to practise. Think about your own workload over the past two weeks and consider how much public health work you currently do. List the public health aspects of your practice.

As you work through the chapter, you will probably want to revisit and revise the list you have developed. You may be surprised to find that you already do a large amount of public health practice. Practice that you might currently consider as quality, audit and holistic care may well be public health practice. By the end of the chapter you may realise that public health is another relevant area of your practice.

Reflective activity

Think about opportunities for expanding the public health dimension of your practice. Read Scenarios 1 and 2 to help trigger your ideas.

Scenario 1

A child sustains a burn injury in the kitchen and is taken to A & E. As well as attending to the burn, the nurse discusses accident prevention and gives some first-aid suggestions to the child and her parents or guardians. Several aspects of this are public health practice. Firstly, the nurse is not limiting her care to the immediate clinical problem, in this case the burn. Rather, she is assessing need using a public health approach by attempting to understand the situation so that she may help to prevent another accident occurring. She is viewing the child as a member of a family and locating her discussion in their specific situation.

If the nurse then developed a display board of information about accident prevention for the waiting area of the A & E department, she would be promoting and protecting the health and well-being of the community in general. In this way, someone not even attending A & E because of a burn caused by a kitchen accident could be alerted to the danger and be more informed about how to avoid it. Developing the public health components of quality and risk management, the nurse might go to a manager and discuss the location of any hot drinks vending machines in the department. Are they located to minimise the potential for scald accidents?

Key phrases

- **Assessing need** – this is the first stage of any intervention with patients, clients or service users.
- **Promoting and protecting health and well-being** – this focuses on health protection, health promotion and the maintenance or restoration of health (Chapter 2).
- **Quality and risk management** – this focuses on quality and risk management in an evidence-based approach to practice.

Scenario 2

A midwife working in a hospital in a disadvantaged area noticed that an increasing number of pregnant women were using drugs. Through gentle, non-accusatory chats with the women, she realised there was a lot of depression and general hopelessness, largely because a local factory had closed down recently, causing massive unemployment. From her chats, the midwife realised that the women felt guilty about taking drugs but they couldn't see any way out of their situation. She asked them what they thought could be done to help and they suggested that it might help if they could talk to other people in a similar situation.

With the women's agreement, the midwife talked to her midwifery colleagues in the community plus the local drug and alcohol misuse team. Working in collaboration and partnership with the women, it was decided to set up drop-in sessions for tea and chat. Over time the women became more confident and less depressed and some were able to stop or minimise their drug-taking. The midwife had played a key role in implementing policy and strategy to improve health and well-being. She had also worked collaboratively to develop a health programme and service to tackle health inequalities.

Key phrases

- **Working in collaboration and partnership** – this means working together not only with users and carers, but also within a multiprofessional and multi-agency arena to better understand or respond to an issue and achieve better care. It is thought that a single organisation cannot understand or contribute to all aspects of care.
- **Implementing policy and strategy** – it is more productive when the practitioner works in partnership with the local community, using their knowledge to devise strategies that will improve health and well-being.
- **Develop a health programme and service to tackle health inequalities** – effective help for disadvantaged groups means giving them access to appropriate services.

Issues in context

All nurses and other health-care practitioners can incorporate public health into their role. Public health tends to be viewed as a limited aspect of nursing practice, but in fact there are many opportunities. If we begin to place the issues in context and think about some of the challenges facing the practitioner, such as a high volume of patients to care for, we could also begin to think of ways to meet these challenges. A limited public health dimension could have been achieved in the two scenarios simply by ensuring that health promotion leaflets were available, which would take little time to organise. But what is needed is a public health perspective on practice, and this public health perspective is often limited or missing in many health-care systems. The focus tends to be very narrow and very individual. The immediate issue is dealt with, but not why the issue arose and whether it can be prevented from recurring. Although it can be difficult to develop a public health approach, it is not impossible.

Over to you

Design a health promotion leaflet to apply to one area of your practice where you know there is a need.

Develop a public health approach to nursing

Developing more of a public health focus may not be as difficult as it first appears, as there are many similarities in the overlap between general nursing practice and public health nursing practice (Figure 3.1). Skills for Health produced the *National Occupational Standards for the Practice of Public Health* to provide a common reference point for practitioners from all the different agencies (health, local authority, voluntary, private) working to reduce inequalities and improve the public's health, so that different practitioners could incorporate them into their own practice settings (Skills for Health 2004). The standards fit into 10 key areas of public health, several of which were covered in the two scenarios. Although public health practice has been categorised into key areas, they do have a common aspect and many nurses will work in two or more key areas at a time. Here are the 10 key areas:

- surveillance and assessment of the population's health and well-being
- promoting and protecting the population's health and well-being
- developing quality and risk management within an evaluative culture
- collaborative working for health
- developing health programmes and services, and reducing inequalities
- policy and strategy development and implementation
- working with and for communities
- strategic leadership for health
- research and development
- ethically managing self, people and resources.

By exploring these areas in more detail, it will become clear how a nurse from any discipline could further develop their public health approach to practice. Notice that public health practice has a lot in common with general nursing practice, including the four stages of assessment, planning priorities, implementing interventions and evaluation. Sometimes, these are separate stages, but generally all four are incorporated into one area of public health practice.

Assess need

All nursing practice involves assessment. But as nursing practice primarily focuses on dealing with illness, there is often little opportunity or requirement to identify need. In many health-care situations a nurse may address a patient's need without consciously assessing or identifying it. For example, a nurse working in a prison health centre may work with prisoners who have long-term mental health problems where the presenting mental ill health issues are treated with medication, but what are the opportunities for improving their health in other ways? Male prisoners may have children and have very little contact with them, which is also contributing to their poor mental health. Could the nurse work with the prison education service to set up a CD-recording service where the prisoners do a talking letter or read a story to their children?

Public health practice differs from general nursing practice in two important ways:

- Assessment of need is never focused solely on the individual.
- Assessment of need is never solely on the here-and-now issues.

When need is identified in a public health context, the process is expanded to consider the individual within a family, within a community and within a wider society; remember the rainbow model from Chapter 2. Consequently, the focus of public health practice may not be an individual but a family or group, a community or population.

Public health practice suits the frustrated detective because it's all about continuing to question and explore the issues. For example, an old man with dementia goes to a day centre for respite three days a week. The service may provide him with useful opportunities for rehabilitation, therapy and good nutrition and give the main carer, his wife, a few hours of relief. This would provide a good service. But a public health approach to need would take other issues into account:

- Is it in the old man's best interests to take him out of his environment?
- Could support be taken into his home?
- What does his wife, the carer, think is the best option for him?
- What are her needs?
- Are there some younger old people in the old man's community who would like to help the old man and his wife on a voluntary basis?

Offering voluntary help might be a useful transition for someone newly retired and wanting to engage more in their local community. They could do this through Crossroads or a similar organisation. It would benefit their own health and put social capital into the community (page 31).

Evidence base

Read about the work of Crossroads at the organisation's website, which also has some case studies.

Evidence base

A social enterprise scheme run by a voluntary sector agency in Liverpool has recently set up a complementary therapy course to pamper exhausted carers for a few hours. They recognise that carers work around the clock and receive very little care for themselves. For further details, visit the *Guardian*'s website.

Plan priorities

Public health practice has a wider focus than general nursing practice and can therefore make a wider contribution to health improvement. Consequently, there may be more choices than usual when prioritising practice. The care provided for an individual user may be restricted to dealing with an urgent need, but that should not prevent a practitioner from doing public health practice. For example, a woman aged 40 with an exacerbation of her chronic rheumatoid arthritis is admitted to hospital for stabilisation. Her 12-year-old daughter visits each day after school and brings along her 6-year-old brother. The nurse notices that the girl looks very tired and she is usually carrying several bags of shopping. A husband or partner never seems to visit. The nurse talks to the woman and discovers that her partner left six months earlier and since then her daughter has been doing a lot of the household jobs.

The woman is very concerned about her daughter, but has no one else she can turn to. With the woman's agreement, the nurse decides to seek help but is unsure where to go. As she knows very little about services outside the hospital, the nurse contacts the hospital social worker. The social worker organises a variety of services to help the family. The nurse feels frustrated that she wasn't able to do more herself and decides to find out how she can give more holistic care. Resource limitations often make it impossible to meet all needs, so it is essential to prioritise aspects of health and well-being to promote and protect.

Over to you

Familiarise yourself and others with agencies in your area that might be able to improve the health of your service users and their carers. These agencies may be public, voluntary or private. You could look in the local phone book, do an internet search, talk to any practitioners from other sectors that come into your practice area, talk to the patient advisory liaison services and the Patients Forum. Set up a database of these services.

Make interventions

Public health interventions may be focused on the individual, the family or the community, and the practitioner may work in a partnership with other agencies. This involves skills such as communication but may also require some knowledge and skill development in areas such as **political awareness** and **enterprise**. For example, during November, nurses in different settings will see injuries caused by fireworks. So in September they could work in partnership with a local fire officer and get an item about the risk of fireworks on local radio or into a local paper. It could explain the

Keywords

Political awareness
Political awareness includes an awareness of health policy and strategy when planning and developing interventions. It also includes knowing which people or committees have influence over different issues, so appropriate messages go to the right people during any initiative

Enterprise
Enterprise involves developing a solution from a business perspective. This may mean that you abandon your usual strategies and try novel and creative ideas

hazards and some simple ways to avoid them. A nurse who does this has demonstrated enterprise and has worked collaboratively and in partnership with other agencies for the health and well-being of the community by helping to reduce the number of firework accidents.

Reflective activity

Think about some of the people you have cared for. Could you have given your practice a greater public health focus by trying some of these interventions?

- Refer the person to a community service
- Liaise with the dietician about the food offered to service users
- Contact the local transport provider about infrequent buses and bus stops that are far from the health service centre
- Compile an evidence base for service change and development

Evaluate the process

If the need is obvious, if the appropriate intervention is clear and if the impact is immediate, then the public health evaluation is similar to many other nursing evaluations. But a public health impact is not always immediate, so the evaluation may differ in several ways. A change in behaviour doesn't usually happen overnight. For example, a 49-year-old man in the coronary care unit may be a smoker and his admission has finally galvanised him into wanting to quit smoking. However, it generally takes several attempts to stop smoking, and the whole process could take years. As a result, we often have to evaluate the 'intermediate indicators of change' (Tones and Tilford 1994), that is, we look for a change in attitude rather than a change in behaviour. The man in the coronary care unit might move from being totally disinterested in quitting smoking to thinking about it and planning how he might do it.

One practitioner alone may not be able to meet all his needs, so might have to refer him to the cardiac rehabilitation nurse or the community smoking cessation adviser. Public health practitioners rarely see the overall outcome of their interventions and this can be frustrating. You often have to be satisfied that you have contributed a piece of the jigsaw or moved someone along the path to better health. It is known colloquially as the drip-drip approach. To adopt the drip-drip approach, you need to understand the cycle of change and locate it in other resources. Chapter 8 covers it in more detail.

> ### *Evidence base*
>
> Go to the website of the National Institute for Health and Clinical Excellence (NICE) and read NICE's draft document on behaviour change.

Public health models for practice

Most nurses and midwives can practise public health. But how do they do it? Public health practice involves many issues and different models that help practitioners delimit the role, the practice agenda and the functions they perform. Public health practice can take many forms. There is a continuum of activity that runs from individual preventive and reactive interventions at one end to population health promotion and proactive interventions at the other. A few practitioners work across the continuum, practitioners such as health visitors, school health advisers and occupational health nurses (SCPHNs), but many contribute to a part of it. Although a practitioner may not actually do it all, a very important public health skill is to know who else is contributing to the continuum of activity. Some of the key factors from a range of models have been simplified and are presented here under the headings preventive, political and participatory.

> ### *Evidence base*
>
> Read Eklan, R., Blair, M. and Robinson, J. A. (2000) Evidence-based practice and health visiting: the need for theoretical underpinnings for evaluation. *Journal of Advanced Nursing*, **31**(6), 1316–1323. This is a useful reference that compares several public health models.
> Visit the Centre for Public Health Excellence's website.

Preventive

The preventive approach is perhaps the most common. It is driven by an epidemiological and medical approach in that need is identified by an understanding of who is at risk of developing a disease. A typical example is a practice nurse who uses cervical cytology to screen people for cervical cancer. Another example is a sexual health adviser who encourages a user with a sexually transmitted infection to inform partners of their potential exposure to the infection.

The preventive model of practice is based on an assumption that people have the opportunity and ability to make rational health choices. But despite the best efforts of the practitioner, this may not always be the case. Remember that the need is often determined by health policy; for example, giving up smoking and tackling obesity are key themes of

Choosing Health (Department of Health 2004a). The service provider has to put these policies into action, and the public health practitioners have to focus on delivering the service that satisfies the policy. The practitioner triggers the patient or service user to begin thinking about the existence of a health need such as a healthier diet and offers assistance in meeting the need.

Evidence base

Several health promotion models explore why people don't always make rational health choices. Read Naidoo, J. and Wills, J. (2001) *Health Studies: An Introduction.* Palgrave, Basingstoke, Hants.

⚷ *Keywords*

Empowerment

To empower someone is to give them power, to enable them to do something or to help them participate. Individual empowerment combines a positive self-image, a sense of control and an ability to influence decisions. Community empowerment is where people and local organisations combine their skills and effort to meet the needs of the community

Political

The political approach departs from a focus dominated by individual choice. It considers how societal or structural factors might influence the way a person makes health choices, factors such as the size of a person's income, the condition of their housing, and whether their community has a lot of crime or drug misuse. As explained in Chapter 2, these issues are closely related to health inequalities and the degree of **empowerment** or enablement felt by individuals and the community. This widens the work of the public health practitioner to include political activity that encourages and supports communities to take action for themselves or where the public health practitioner works as an advocate for individuals and communities.

Another political approach is to review and develop services such as new roles or service provision after a health needs assessment reveals gaps in provision. The political model acknowledges the diversity of need in a particular area and responds with appropriate services. For example, peer educators may be trained by public health practitioners to work with people from their own community. Women who have breastfed successfully might be recruited to learn how to support other women wanting to breastfeed. Similarly, people with long-term conditions such as diabetes are using their expertise to help others. Peer education is highly successful, particularly in communities where people may be reluctant to work with professionals.

Evidence base

Go to the Improvement Network's website and read the article that explains how peer educators helped to build community partnerships in the East Midlands.

Participatory

In the participatory approach, the user has a much stronger role in all aspects of care, be it identifying need, prioritising actions, deciding on appropriate solutions or deciding on what has worked. It is distinguished by the fact that power is more equitably distributed between all parties involved, so that no one person is seen to have the deciding vote in a situation; it is much more democratic. It recognises that professionals have a knowledge base, but it also recognises that users and carers are often experts on their health, their needs and their situation, and they often have a better knowledge of the issues than the practitioners who work with them. The participatory approach encourages users and carers to know and feel that their contribution is wanted, respected and relevant. This might be quite new for people who have only experienced relationships where the health-care provider is the dominant partner that offers standard solutions with little choice or negotiation.

Evidence base

Revisit the summary of *Our Health, Our Care, Our Say* at the Department of Health's website.

How to combine public health models

The practice situation or context will significantly influence the choice of public health model. A single model may be appropriate for some situations but other situations will probably require a combination of models, although one model may be more dominant than the others (Figure 3.2). Returning to the old man cared for by his wife, introduced on page 41, let's suppose he attends the unit for respite care three days per week. The nurse talks to his wife, who is reluctant to leave him as she feels she knows her husband and his needs better than anyone else. But the nurse senses that his wife is weary and suggests that she too attends the unit on some days as there are services such as hairdressing and activities such as cards, bingo and trips to the seaside. After the wife says yes, the nurse approaches the managers who will make the arrangements. The nurse worked through all three public health models – preventive, participatory and political – to achieve the best outcome for users and carers.

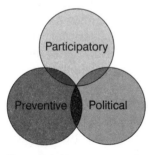

Figure 3.2 How to combine public health models

Preventive

The nurse takes a proactive approach by looking to see how else the carer's health could be improved beyond the provision of three days' respite from a caring role. One of the appropriate interventions was to expand the respite service to include the wife. A preventive model would still have been used if the nurse had advised the carer about routine health surveillance available at the GP practice, encouraged uptake of flu immunisation and made the carer aware of other support services in the area. The key message is that care is not necessarily limited to the initial need for referral, but the nurse is searching for other health needs and endeavours to stimulate an awareness of health needs in the carer.

Participatory

The nurse tries to adopt a partnership relationship with user and carer, the old man and his wife. Although the nurse cares for the user three days a week, she also tries to engage with him as a man who lives with his wife and as a member of a community. She therefore sees the respite service as acting in partnership with the wife, the family and other informal or formal support services that help to manage their health and illness. There is a suggestion box with pens and comment cards inside the entrance to the respite care unit. The nurse encourages users and carers to post their opinions and comments about the service: what is good, what could be improved and suggestions for further developments. Every two months she displays a notice beside the suggestion box that shows what suggestions were made and how the unit responded.

The nurse is using the suggestion box to help develop a plan of action to respond to the assessed needs of carers. She invites some carers and users to be involved in the decision-making process, she encourages them to speak their thoughts and she encourages them to post suggestions in the suggestion box. For example, she finds out whether users are happy that relatives spend time with them in the day unit. The day unit is primarily to provide respite care, so the users must be the priority. If, during discussions, the users had rejected the idea of open access to carers, the nurse could have tried to find a different way to address the carer's needs. And if the new solution caused the nurse to deviate from her main service provision, she may well have been blocked by her managers.

Political

The nurse is aware of the policy to encourage greater participation and involvement in care (Department of Health 1999, 2000, 2001, 2003, 2004b, 2006b), so she realises this is something the NHS trust must work towards. Therefore managers would probably view this as efficient practice. Before initiating the suggestion box in the unit, the nurse had discussions with management to see whether they would support it. She also set up a communication system with management of two 30-minute meetings each month for sharing the suggestions and action planning. Before her meeting on opening up the unit to carers, the nurse produced a proposal that covered these items:

● Find out how many carers may be invited to attend at a time to comply with health and safety requirements.

- A carer will draw up a rota for the visits, so the unit can determine the visiting days, the frequency and whether visits create extra work for the nursing staff.
- Would the catering manager be willing to supply extra meals for carers?
- Would one of the carers deliver the collective payment for the meals to the staff canteen towards the end of the afternoon?
- It is very expensive to transport patients to the centre. The region has free travel for people over 60. Perhaps relatives could make their own way to and from the day unit. The volunteer transport service could also be contacted.

Evidence base

Read Section 11 of the Health and Social Care Act 2001. Section 11 is on patient and public involvement.

Public health skills

To show you the skills needed to practise public health, Table 3.1 summarises some generic skills aligned to the 10 key areas of public health practice. There is a long list of competencies for public health practice (Skills for Health 2004) and a long list of proficiencies for SCPHNs (Nursing and Midwifery Council 2004a), but they are not listed here.

Table 3.1 Key areas and key skills of public health practice

Key areas	Key skills
Surveillance and assessment	Assessing need
Promoting and protecting health and well-being	Working in partnership
Developing quality and risk management	Preventing or minimising harm
Collaborative working	Raising awareness
Developing health programmes and services	Project working
Policy and strategy development and implementation	Implementing policy
Working with and for communities	Supporting and enabling
Strategic leadership	Leading and managing
Research and development	Practising evidence-based practice
Ethically managing self and others	Managing ethically and effectively

Evidence base

Go to the Skills for Health website for more detail and to see the individual public health competencies.

In 2004 the NMC organised the 10 key areas of public health practice into four domains to enable SCPHNs on the third part of the NMC register to undertake public health work with a clear focus on the process and outcome. Go to the NMC's website for more detail and to see the standards of proficiency.

Whether a nurse or health-care practitioner is assessing the health or well-being of individuals, groups or communities through needs identification (health needs assessment), raising awareness in a partnership approach for health and well-being, or doing a project to develop health programmes and services, they will not be effective without the vitally important core skills that underpin public health practice: communication skills, interpersonal skills and therapeutic intervention skills. This means more than being able to pass on health promotion information. In many public health interventions the individual, group or community may not have articulated a health issue. The skill of the nurse or health-care practitioner is to engage with the individual or group, help them to see that they have a health need, then encourage them to do something about it or, if necessary, to act as an advocate. The case study below shows how the skills, the models and the key areas come together in good public health practice.

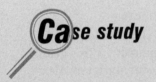 **Case study**

Katy and Alex

Tom is a staff nurse on a paediatric unit in a busy general hospital. He is concerned about Katy, mother of Alex, an 8-year-old boy recently diagnosed with diabetes. Tom was on duty when Alex was diagnosed and remembers how difficult Katy had found it. Two months later, Alex has been readmitted to adjust his insulin requirement. Tom thinks that Katy is depressed as she doesn't seem as chatty and inquisitive as before.

Alex seems to be making good progress in coping with his diabetes. Tom decides to see if he can find out the problem with Katy. While Alex is in the hospital classroom, Tom initiates a conversation with Katy and asks how things are going. Katy says everything is fine, but Tom senses that is far from the truth and gently begins to talk about how difficult it can be when something unexpected happens. Without mentioning names, Tom gives examples of other families who have struggled with their child's diagnosis. Soon Katy bursts into tears. She begins to tell Tom how guilty she feels that it might be her fault as she had a sugar craving in pregnancy. She fears that her thoughtless actions could mean that her son ends up as a blind amputee.

Tom listens carefully to all Katy says, occasionally paraphrasing her words to check he has understood her correctly. When she has finished, Tom begins to explain that Katy's feelings are normal and that many people in similar situations have expressed similar feelings. Tom asks Katy what she thinks she may need to help her through this difficult time. Katy seems too upset to think clearly, so Tom begins to tell her about a support group he set up for parents to help each other cope with having a diabetic

continued

child. After meeting monthly for six months in the hospital with Tom and other people, such as a specialist diabetes nurse, a dietician, someone from Diabetes UK and a social worker, the group decided to meet outside the hospital in a local community hall.

Tom thinks he has given enough information for the moment but invites Katy to go along to the group, meet its members and hear more about it. Katy doesn't feel like going to the group, so Tom suggests that someone from the group could come and see her while Alex is in hospital. Katy says she would like that.

- What other indications might show that Katy is depressed?
- How might Tom have phrased questions to encourage Katy to open up?

Tom worked through the combined preventive, participatory and political model. He was preventing mental ill health with all its possible ramifications. He worked in a participatory way with Katy to determine what she thought was the best course of action. He showed his political influence when he set up the group.

We can also see the 10 key areas of public health practice as separate units or as overlapping and interconnecting with the issues running throughout. For example, at any stage, Tom could have completed his intervention with Katy and he would still have been contributing to the public health approach, but instead he continued through to a conclusion. Tom worked along the whole continuum of public health skills. Moreover, a key issue in the case study was working in partnership and collaboration not only with Katy, but also with other services and agencies to deliver the support group. Let's look at how Tom worked through the 10 key areas of public health practice using public health skills:

- **Surveillance and assessment** – Tom used his skills of identifying need to assess Katy's health and well-being and indirectly Alex's health and well-being, as a depressed mother would have an impact on Alex.
- **Promoting and protecting health and well-being** – Tom protected the health and well-being of Katy and Alex. Working in partnership, Tom helped Katy see that what she was going through was normal.
- **Developing quality and risk management** – Tom realised that a depressed mother could have disastrous consequences for herself and Alex, so Tom was preventing or reducing the risk of harm.
- **Collaboratively working for health** – Tom was working with Katy to raise her awareness of her needs.
- **Developing health programmes and services** – Tom was instrumental in setting up the project to develop a support group.
- **Policy and strategy development and implementation** – Tom was implementing the policy of the 'expert patient' by setting up a group.

- **Working with and for communities** – Tom had worked with a community of people who had needs associated with diabetes and enabled and encouraged them to form a group.
- **Strategic leadership for health** – Tom employed leadership skills to develop the group.
- **Research and development** – Tom was working within an evidence base that suggests users are often experts in their conditions and can learn more from each other than from professionals.
- **Ethically managing self and others** – Tom was managing himself and others, ethically and effectively working within the Code of Professional Conduct (Nursing and Midwifery Council 2004b).

However, the most important skills that led to a positive outcome were Tom's core skills: his communication skills, interpersonal skills and therapeutic intervention skills. Tom sensed that something was troubling Katy. He needed to find out tactfully and diplomatically what was bothering her. His approach was gentle but assertive, and by using open-ended questions, listening carefully, paraphrasing and normalising the situation, his intuitive approach enabled the beginning of a therapeutic process to prevent mental health problems that could have affected Katy plus Alex and the wider family.

Figure 3.3 combines all the areas of public health practice, the public health models and public health skills in this chapter to create a framework for a public health approach to nursing practice. At the core of the framework is the user or group, which could be individuals, families, communities or populations, or a combination of these. Each of the circles contains issues you must consider when you adopt a public health approach to practice. Here are some questions that should be asked by the nurse or health-care practitioner:

- Which model – preventive, political or participatory – or which combination of models will guide the parameters of practice?
- Which of the 10 key areas of public health practice will be drawn on?
- Which of the public health skills will be required?
- Which core skills will be required? The core skills are communication skills, interpersonal skills and therapeutic intervention skills.

Notice that the framework is presented in a circular design. This reinforces the notion that public health practice does not have a clear beginning or end; indeed there is always a public health need to be addressed. Also notice that the lines between the circles are not solid but dashed. This indicates that in a public health approach to practice there is always the potential for movement between the circles as you develop your understanding of need and responses. Referring back to spheres of practice on page 37, there is also a clear message that with any nursing or health-care role there is the potential to locate practice at different points in the framework at different times depending on need and

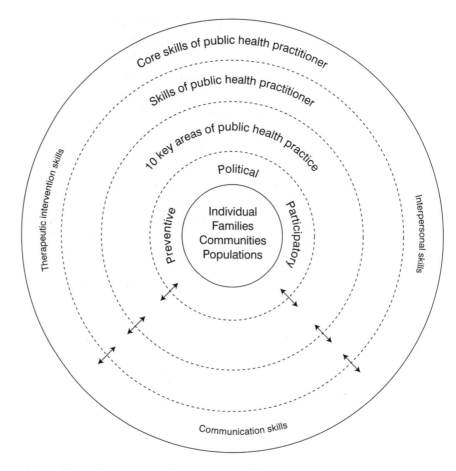

Figure 3.3 A framework for a public health approach to nursing practice. See Table 3.1 for the key areas and key skills

context. It also emphasises the message that a public health approach to practice is seldom confined to the efforts of one practitioner but requires working in partnership with other people and agencies. Scrutinising the framework helps practitioners to identify their contribution to the overall process and to see the roles of other practitioners.

Conclusion

This chapter has unpacked the meaning of public health approaches to nursing and health-care practice. It has encouraged you to examine your practice to see how you already contribute to public health, and it has invited you to think about how much more you could do. It has used scenarios and case studies to demystify the theory behind public health practice and it has looked at different approaches based on key areas of practice, models and skills. Having read this chapter, you can now begin to think about how to develop the knowledge and skills needed for public health practice.

RRRRRapid recap

Check your progress so far by working through each of the following questions.

1. What are the similarities between general nursing practice and public health practice?
2. Name the three main models of public health practice.
3. List three core skills that are common to public health practice and nursing or health-care practice.
4. List five generic public health skills.

If you have difficulty with more than one of the questions, read through the section again to refresh your understanding before moving on.

References

Department of Health (1999) *Patient and Public Involvement in the New NHS*. HMSO, London.

Department of Health (2000) *The NHS Plan*. HMSO, London.

Department of Health (2001) *Health and Social Care Act: Patient and Public Involvement*. HMSO, London.

Department of Health (2003) *Strengthening Accountability: Involving Patients and the Public*. HMSO, London.

Department of Health (2004a) *Choosing Health: Making Healthier Choices Easier*. HMSO, London.

Department of Health (2004b) *The NHS Improvement Plan: Putting People at the Heart of Public Services*. HMSO, London.

Department of Health (2006a) *Our Health, Our Care, Our Say*. HMSO, London.

Department of Health (2006b) *A Stronger Local Voice*. HMSO, London.

Eklan, R., Blair, M. and Robinson, J. A. (2000) Evidence-based practice and health visiting: the need for theoretical underpinnings for evaluation. *Journal of Advanced Nursing*, **31**(6), 1316–1323.

Naidoo, J. and Wills, J. (2001) *Health Studies: An Introduction*. Palgrave, Basingstoke, Hants.

Nursing and Midwifery Council (2004a) *Standards of Proficiency for Specialist Community Public Health Nurses*. NMC, London.

Nursing and Midwifery Council (2004b) *The NMC Code of Professional Conduct*. NMC, London.

Skills for Health (2004) *National Occupational Standards for the Practice of Public Health*. Skills for Health, Bristol.

Tones, K. and Tilford, S. (1994) *Health Education: Education, Effectiveness and Equity*. Chapman & Hall, London.

4

Assessing health needs

Jan Mitcheson

Learning outcomes

By the end of the chapter you should be able to:

★ Understand the concept of need

★ Understand the range of perspectives used to define need

★ Identify the process of health needs assessment

★ Select from a range of HNA tools.

Introduction

Since the NHS and Community Care Act 1990, successive government policies have consistently emphasised the importance of delivering services in response to identified needs (Department of Health 2005, 2006). Assessing the health needs of individuals, groups and communities is the fundamental basis of public health practice and is the starting point for using a public health approach in your practice area. A health needs assessment (HNA) is a systematic way of determining the needs of your patients, service users or community and will help inform the service you deliver. HNAs can be used to validate the populations currently in need of services and to identify new populations with unmet needs (Petersen and Alexander 2001).

The concept of need

Definitions of need are contentious and open to various interpretations. There has been significant debate over the meaning and nature of 'need'. Orr (1992) suggested that need is social because it is defined according to the standards of society, relative in that it will vary from age to age and community to community, and evaluative in that it is based on value judgements. It is also claimed that need is socially constructed and closely bound up with personal identities, expectation and context (Cowley 2002). Several types of need exist but all can usually be defined in terms of some kind of discrepancy between a desired state and an actual state. Bradshaw's much quoted taxonomy has four types of need (Bradshaw 1972).

Bradshaw's four types of need

Felt need

Felt need is need that is perceived by an individual or a community. Bradshaw (1994) considered it to be an inadequate measure of 'real need' as it relies on individual perceptions. People might not know that they are in need of a service or may not wish to acknowledge to themselves or others that they are in need.

Expressed need

Expressed need is a felt need translated into action, sometimes known as a demand. Expressed need is commonly used by health planners to give an indication of the amount of need for a service, such as waiting lists. Bradshaw says it too is an inadequate measure of real need as many people have felt needs but do not have the resources to express those needs to others or are too frightened to express them (Bradshaw 1994).

Normative need

Normative needs are needs defined by a professional or expert. A professional association determines a standard. For example, the British Dietetic Association sets nutritional standards; if a person falls short of that standard, they are said to be in need.

Comparative need

Comparative need is determined by comparing two groups of people with similar characteristics where one group receives a service and the other group does not receive that service. Suppose women in area A require treatment for infertility and do not receive it, then they are in need compared with women in area B who do receive it. This is a relatively simple example and needs are rarely as clear cut as this implies, but it does illustrate the point. Comparative need is about 'equity', equal provision for equal need. Recent high-profile cases on drug therapy for breast cancer have challenged decisions by primary care trusts (PCTs) on how to distribute finite resources.

Map of unmet needs

A map of unmet needs may be more relevant to contemporary society. The idea emerged from a recent report prepared by the Young Foundation (Buonfino and Geissendorfer 2006) for the Commission for Unclaimed Assets. Using a wide range of **quantitative** and **qualitative data**, the authors were able to identify and map the most pressing unmet needs of the population of Britain. The report highlighted four main categories of need (Table 4.1) and identified 40 key needs in six clusters (Table 4.2).

⚷ *Keywords*

Quantitative data
Quantitative data focuses on numbers and frequencies

Qualitative data
Qualitative data emphasises meaning and experience

Evidence base

Go to the Young Foundation's website and read the report by Buonfino and Geissendorfer. You will find it very helpful in understanding the broader definition of need.

Table 4.1 Needs divided into four main categories

Category of need	Description
Physical needs and resources	Basic needs for health, shelter, food and reproduction. Lack of these items can bring considerable harm to a person, ranging from homelessness to illness
Needs for skills and capabilities	Skills and aptitudes needed to take part in society and exercise freedom. Lack of these skills often leads to other kinds of need
Need for care and advice	Care, advice, nurture and support, plus the need for others
Psychic needs	Related needs for love, recognition, understanding and happiness

Table 4.2 Forty needs grouped into six clusters

Factor	Description
Poverty	Groups suffering from classic poverty of power, money and place: poor people, elderly people, people with disabilities, people with mental illnesses, single parents
Destitution	People who fall through the cracks of public policy caused by globalisation: asylum seekers, trafficked people, modern slaves, undocumented migrants, etc.
Fractured families	People whose needs arise from fractured families and who cannot benefit from family support: people leaving care and having no one to rely on, overstretched parents. People from weak family substitutes that fail to provide the necessary care and support
Psychic	People whose needs relate less to material things and poverty, but more to anxiety and stress due to a changing and more demanding working life, family breakdowns, loneliness, isolation, etc.
Damaging consumption	People whose needs are the result of prosperity, success, globalisation and better spending power. They have improved lifestyles, life chances and medical care but they suffer from a rise in chronic and infectious diseases, bad diet, STDs, etc.
Violence and abuse	The passive victims of violence, road accidents, crime and abuse

Health needs assessment

Some definitions

Some definitions of leadership are given below:

> the capacity to benefit from health care – the greater the ability to benefit, the greater is the need – it is the effectiveness of the treatment rather than the severity of the illness which determine a person's need
>
> Stevens and Gabby (1991)

> a process of measuring ill health of a population
>
> Pickin and Leger (1994)

> a need for health care can be said to exist when an individual has a condition for which there are effective and suitable interventions
>
> Hooper and Longworth (2002)

> a description of those factors which must be addressed in order to improve the health of the population
>
> Billings (2002)

> a systematic method for reviewing the health issues facing a population, leading to agreed priorities and resource allocation that will improve health and reduce inequalities
>
> Cavanagh and Chadwick (2005)

Reflective activity

Take a moment to think about the definitions.

- What are the key differences in these definitions?
- What might be the difficulties of defining health needs in terms of effectiveness of interventions?
- What do these definitions say about how we view health?

⊶ᴨ *Keywords*

Effectiveness
The extent to which interventions have achieved their goals

We require a broader definition of HNA than some of these definitions. It is unhelpful to see health needs only as problems or diseases that are amenable to treatment. Needs assessment is not the same as measuring clinical **effectiveness**. The key difference is that individuals, communities and populations have health needs whereas interventions are assessed on effectiveness. The proper focus for HNA must be on identifying the needs of the population that are important to them and that must be addressed in order to tackle inequalities and bring about improved health.

Key perspectives on HNA

The different definitions of HNA arise from the different theoretical and ethical perspectives that underpin the approaches to HNA. Here are the four principal perspectives:

- epidemiological perspective
- sociological perspective
- economic perspective
- consumer perspective.

Epidemiological perspective

Chapter 2 defined epidemiology as a population science that focuses on the study of the distribution, frequency and determinants of health and disease in the population. Epidemiologists consider HNA as largely about the collection of data in relation to mortality (lives lost) and morbidity (amount of ill health in a community) plus the associated risks of cause and effect. Population data such as age, ethnicity and socio-economic profiles helps to identify patterns of ill health related to specific groups in a community or practice area. This approach is a fundamental and important part of the public health practice and is widely used in public health departments. But epidemiology depends on accurate, complete and timely data, which is often difficult to obtain and is insufficient for determining needs. Chapter 5 has a full discussion of the advantages and limitations of an epidemiological perspective.

Sociological perspective

The sociological perspective views health and social needs as interdependent and argues that the concept of need is too complex to be quantified merely in epidemiological terms. Poverty is identified as a key element related to ill health. Sociologists, among others, argue persuasively that if health inequalities are to be reduced and the gap narrowed between the health of upper and lower social classes, then material deprivation is central to any process that aims to identify need (Acheson 1998; Wanless 2004).

Economic perspective

Health economics developed in the late 1960s and examines the allocation and distribution of resources. It uses the key concept of efficiency as a criterion for allocating finite resources to obtain maximum health improvement. Many health economists subscribe to the view that, in their terms, HNA exercises avoid the difficult and demanding choices in delivering health care, such as which services to deliver, which patients should be offered services and which patients should be refused services. They argue that it is not sufficient to collect data and information about health needs and allocate resources accordingly, as there are also very difficult moral choices to make about whether to meet one need or another. Now this may seem extreme and somewhat divorced from the world of the nurse or public health practitioner, but in every situation individual practitioners have to decide how much of their time – a scarce resource – they can give to one person or one group of people, often instead of giving it to a different person or a different group of people. In that sense, HNA inevitably produces some form of rationing (Newdick 2005).

The economic perspective says there is a dynamic relationship between need, supply and demand (Figure 4.1). Its proponents claim that it relies on quantifying demand, indicating value for money and establishing the effectiveness of health-care interventions; they say this makes it an objective and valid method. Health economists have undoubtedly contributed to the HNA debate by pointing out that it costs money to meet people's needs and insisting that we investigate the relative costs of meeting different needs (Robinson and Elkan 1996). Quality-adjusted life years (**QALYs**) are frequently used by health economists as a tool to measure the outcomes or benefits of interventions.

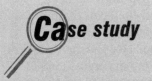

Keywords

QALYs

Quality-adjusted life years: to calculate QALYs, multiply estimated length of life by estimated quality of life from the service user's perspective

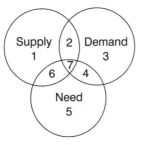

Figure 4.1 Venn diagram of supply, need and demand

1 *Supply that is neither demanded nor needed*
2 *Demand that is supplied but not needed*
3 *Demand that is not needed and not supplied*
4 *Demand that is needed but not supplied*
5 *Need that is not demanded and not supplied*
6 *Need that is supplied but not demanded*
7 *Need that is demanded and supplied*

Case study

Mrs Smith and granddaughter

Mrs Smith is 80 years old and has been experiencing severe pain in her left hip for some time. She has been diagnosed as requiring a hip replacement but has been told that she will have to wait six months before the operation can be done at her local hospital. At the same time, her granddaughter, aged 7, is having an operation to put grommets in her ears, even though evidence suggests this may not be best practice.

● Mrs Smith and her granddaughter, do they each have a need?

● Is there a demand?

● Is there a service supplied to meet their need?

● What does this mean for Mrs Smith and her granddaughter?

QALYs can be estimated for an individual, group or population. Their main advantage is that they provide a common unit of comparison for outcomes from diverse health-care interventions (Powell 2003). But there are some well-documented difficulties in this approach (Bowling 2004; Mooney 2003). There are methodological concerns about estimating survival and there are ethical concerns about how quality of life in illness can be measured and how different health states should be valued.

Consumer perspective

Government policy over the past decade has placed increasing emphasis on ensuring that services are designed, developed and delivered in consultation with the people who use them, the consumers (Department of Health 2005). There is now a requirement to improve **community engagement** and give the public a stronger voice in the commissioning process, particularly when developing new services. Furthermore, the government (Department of Health 2006) has opened the doors to greater choice and competition in the provision of services, particularly services from providers traditionally outside the mainstream NHS, such as voluntary, charitable and community organisations.

○━π *Keywords*

Community engagement
The process of involving key stakeholders in communities, in the prioritisation and development of services. It includes consultation and working in partnership with statutory organisations

Summary

A range of theoretical perspectives underpin HNA. It is doubtful whether people will reach a consensus on the exact nature of HNA. The challenge for nurses and other public health practitioners is to combine the benefits of all four perspectives to get a comprehensive picture of the health needs in the target population or community. The next section considers some guiding principles to help achieve it.

HNA principles

Remember that patterns of need change over time. HNA is not an end in itself, but a means of using information to help plan your service delivery. It cannot and should not be a single activity in terms of time, perspective or completion. HNA is a complex, ongoing process that takes skill to accomplish (Cowley 2000). If it becomes too mechanistic or too structured, if it overemphasises form-filling or data collection, it is in danger of not addressing the needs that are important to the public (Mitcheson and Cowley 2003). HNA is about making sense of people's complex and difficult situations. When determining and understanding the health needs of the people, it is so important that you meet and work with them on their own, in their family or in their community.

HNA purposes

- To search for and raise awareness of needs.
- To identify the pattern of health and illness and health inequality.

- To set priorities, influence policies and target unmet needs.
- To plan appropriate interventions and services.
- To enable efficient and effective ways of using scarce resources to maximise the benefits of health care.

How to do an HNA

There are tools and resources to help you do an HNA. Whichever method you choose, produce a thorough plan that has clear goals and objectives; sets appropriate timeframes; identifies appropriate interventions, key responsibilities and resources; and has a means of evaluation. The Health Development Agency (2004) has published a very useful five-step guide developed from the original work of Hooper and Longworth (2002). It is available on the NICE website. Figure 4.2 shows the five steps.

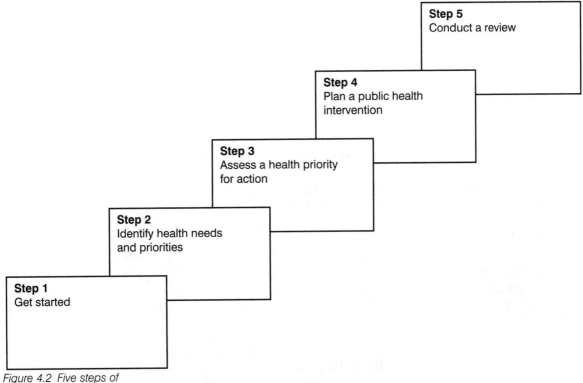

Step 5
Conduct a review

Step 4
Plan a public health intervention

Step 3
Assess a health priority for action

Step 2
Identify health needs and priorities

Step 1
Get started

Figure 4.2 Five steps of health needs assessment

Step 1 Get started: ask these questions

What population and why?

Have a clear idea of the target population from the outset. It could be a group of people with a specific disease or condition, a specific client group or people who use a particular service. It may be easier to get a clear picture if you work in a specific area and have already identified a number of priorities. If you are working in primary care or some other community setting, you will probably want to know more about the community in which you work. In that sense, HNA is not just about the individual needs of your patients or client group but is more likely to be about the needs of the wider population or community. In the rest of this chapter, the terms 'group' or 'community' are used to refer to the target population.

What am I trying to achieve?

You need to be very clear about the aims and objectives of your HNA and set the parameters for your work – what you can and can't do. This will set the direction for your work and ensure it stays on track.

Who needs to be involved?

HNA is not a one-person endeavour and you will need to develop robust partnerships with other people who are interested in the project. Remember that it's about the collective effort and that you will need a range of skills and expertise plus loads of enthusiasm. Appoint a strong leader and have at least one person who will make sure the job gets done.

What resources do I need?

Consider the resources you will need to complete your HNA. Be clear about the timeframe for your work.

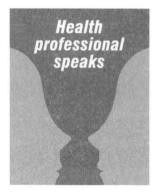

Health professional speaks

Public health nurse
Identifying why you are doing this health needs assessment, who you are doing it for and who and what you need to help you is the best way of ensuring that you achieve what you want.

Over to you

From your experience, choose a group or community that you wish to work with. Use the four key questions to sketch out your HNA:

- What population and why?
- What am I trying to achieve?
- Who needs to be involved?
- What resources do I need?

⊙━ᴋ *Keywords*

Population or community profiling

Population or community profiling is about gathering information on a specific group, population or community and from several different perspectives

Step 2 Identify health needs and priorities

Gather data that will help you identify the health needs of your target population. This is often called **population or community profiling**. The development of a profile that uses multiple sources of data allows you to build a comprehensive picture of the health needs of a population (Billings 2002). Each source or method that you use can give you a different piece of the jigsaw. Create a jigsaw with enough pieces so you can see the whole picture but not too many pieces so it becomes tedious and you don't complete it. It is vital to involve local people and service users to get a true picture of their needs. Chapter 5 contains more guidance on the required types of data and how to interpret them.

Frameworks for gathering data

⊙━ᴋ *Keywords*

Participatory rapid appraisal

A team gathers data about the needs and resources of a particular population or community from a variety of sources, including the community itself

There are several frameworks to help gather information for HNA. Some will be more useful than others; it depends on the work you do. One approach is **participatory rapid appraisal** (Figure 4.3).

Participatory rapid appraisal

Health policy — Local and national		
Educational services	**Health services** Types of provision, access, user views	**Social services** Services available
Physical environment Housing and public amenities	**Socio-economic environment** Employment	**Disease and disability** Type and amount
Community composition Age, gender, social class and levels of deprivation	**Community organisation and structure** Transport networks and boundaries	**Community capacity** Assets and resources

Figure 4.3 Participatory rapid appraisal

Rapid appraisal has recently become more popular in the UK, guided by the work of Annett and Rifkin (1996) and Murray (1999). Rapid appraisal is useful as it gathers a significant amount of data in a short time (2 weeks) and involves community participation. It is based on the health for all (HFA) philosophy of the World Health Organization (WHO), which emphasises equity, participation and collaboration. Information is gathered for each block of the pyramid to give a multifaceted picture of the needs. It pays particular attention to the assets and resources the community has already accrued plus the problems it has encountered. Data is collected in three ways:

- existing data from official sources, such as the Office for National Statistics (ONS)
- focus group interviews with key informants, such as individuals with knowledge of the community because of their job or social standing
- observations and written documents about the community.

The data is used to assemble a pyramid that describes the community's problems and priorities. Success depends on building a planning process that rests on a strong base of community information (Murray 1999).

Murray (1999) outlines how this approach has been adapted to practice and used successfully in three different ways. In the first study, an expanded primary care team identified the needs of 1,200 residents on a small housing estate in central Edinburgh. The second study looked at the same population but focused on the mental health needs of the population. In the third study, three community mental health nurses used the approach to familiarise themselves with the area and assess the need for new services.

The method has been applied in several different ways and in a variety of settings; Lazenbatt and McMurray (2004) used the tool to assess women's psychosocial needs in a deprived inner-city area of Northern Ireland. Pepall *et al.* (2007) used it to assess the needs of a rural Balinese village.

Rapid appraisal has great potential and seems to work best on a small homogeneous group. If you are working with a group of patients or service users with a specific condition, you may find that rapid appraisal is an appropriate method. It does have some important limitations plus the appraising team have to invest considerable time and train thoroughly in gathering data and leading focus groups.

Evidence base

Download the information pyramid from the BMJ website.

Reflective activity

Think about the target group or community that you wish to focus on then use the participatory rapid appraisal framework to answer these questions:

- How many people are in your target population?
- Where are they located?
- What data is currently available for them?
- What are their common experiences?
- How does the target group or target community perceive its needs?
- How can you reach those who might not normally engage with your service?

Windshield survey components

To get a quick initial sense and feel of the community in which you work, Stanhope and Lancaster (2004) suggest a windshield assessment using the format in Table 4.3. Take public transport, walk or have someone drive you while you take notes of what you see. The windshield survey is organised into elements with specific questions related to each element. Visit the area once during the day and once in the evening; it may be advisable not to go alone. This is a useful approach if you are new to working in a geographical community and want to get an initial assessment of the needs of that community. It gives you an opportunity to observe the community in several dimensions. Besides observing an area, gauge what the community is like from the people that live there. Take time to talk with the community leaders and other influential people, such as local councillors or church leaders, but above all, talk to the residents to find out what's really happening.

Table 4.3 Format for a windshield assessment

Element	Questions
Housing	How old are the houses? What is the architecture? What materials are they built from? Are they owned privately, by a local authority or by a housing association? What is their general condition? Are there signs of disrepair, broken windows, etc.? What type of heating is available?
Open space	How much open space is there and what is its quality? Are there lawns, flower beds or trees?
Boundaries	Where does the community begin and end? Are the boundaries natural, such as rivers and roads, or enforced, such as economic and industrial? Does the community have a name, official or otherwise?
Public areas	Where are the hang-out areas? For what groups and at what hours? Is there a sense of territorialism or are they open to everyone?
Transport	How do people get around? By car, by bus, by bike or on foot? Are the streets and roads conducive to good transportation? How frequent is public transport?
Services	Are there social services, doctors, dentists, recreation centres, cinemas, parks and estate agents? Are they in use or boarded up?
Shops	Where do people shop? Are there local shops or out-of-town stores? Is there a market?
People	Who do you see around? Is there a police presence? Do you see anyone you would not expect? What animals do you see? Are there stray cats and dogs or guard dogs?
Signs of decay	Is the area on the way up or on the way down? Is it alive? How would you decide? Is there rubbish on the streets? Are there abandoned cars? Are there posters for community activities, meetings, etc.?

Table 4.3 Format for a windshield assessment (continued)

Element	Questions
Religion	What is the predominant religion? What denomination are the churches and other places of worship? Does the church have a presence in the community?
Race and ethnicity	Is the area integrated? What is the predominant language? Are there food stores?
Health and morbidity	What evidence do you see of acute or chronic disease, alcoholism, drug use, mental health issues? How far is the nearest hospital, clinic or surgery?
Media	What form of media is most important to your community?

Adapted from Stanhope and Lancaster (2004)

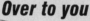

Over to you

Make a list of the strengths and limitations of rapid appraisal and the windshield survey. Then decide which is more appropriate for your HNA?

Other tools

HNA often lacks an assessment of how the community can help to remedy problems or inequalities. But there are now tools that you can use with the community to determine the capacity of the community to organise and participate in public health activities. Surveys are used to highlight existing local organisations and the potential to move forward. This approach values the skills and talents of groups and specifically asks about achievements. It is particularly useful for engaging with groups that don't normally engage with more formal processes of consultation.

Evidence base

Read Skinner, S. and Wilson, M. (2005) *Assessing Community Strengths: A Practical Handbook for Planning Capacity Building*. Community Development Foundation, London. It describes the community strength assessment approach used in Bradford.

Making sense of the data

Collecting data may be time-consuming, but in many ways it is the easy part of HNA. The tricky part is making sense of the data you have collected. Billings (2002) used Yin's (1994) case study design to develop a useful method that assembles data from a variety of sources and observes the patterns or themes that emerge. When you have finished your data analysis, you will probably find a range of issues that need to be tackled. Choosing the highest-priority issue is a central aspect of HNA and depends on several factors. Cavanagh and Chadwick (2005) offer a pragmatic approach and suggest impact (Table 4.4) and changeability (Table 4.5) as criteria for prioritising issues:

- **Impact** – a high impact exists when a significant number of people are affected. Perhaps the number of teenage pregnancies in your area is above the national average.
- **Changeability** – high changeability exists when it is possible to do something about the causes of the health condition. For high numbers of teenage pregnancies this could be teaching negotiation skills in schoolchildren – how to say no to sex – or providing drop-in services to increase the availability of information and condoms.

Table 4.4 How to set out an impact assessment

Health condition and determinant	Severity of impact			Number of people affected per year
	High: can definitely change	Medium: some aspects can be changed	Low: cannot be changed or unknown	

Table 4.5 How to set out a changeability assessment

Health condition and determinant	Level of prevention, ranked from 0 (lowest) to 10 (highest)			
	Primary: prevents the problem occurring	Secondary: prevents the problem progressing	Tertiary: prevents consequences or complications of the problem	Score*

*Higher scores indicate increased likelihood of changeability

Cavanagh and Chadwick (2005) suggest that the following questions are then asked to determine the priorities:

- Are there relevant professional/organisational guidelines/policies that recommend action?
- Are your priorities national and local priorities?
- Does your list of changeable priorities address inequalities?

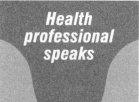

Health visitor
We thought we had a very good idea about the health needs of our community until we worked with the community on the HNA. What they thought was a priority was very different to what we thought

Step 3 Assess a health priority for action

Determine what action you can take to address the priorities you identified in Step 2. This will help you to implement an effective, acceptable and feasible intervention. Most published work points to the National Institute for Health and Clinical Effectiveness (NICE) as an authoritative source of what works well, but more creative solutions to health issues can be found within your community. Always explore ways to strengthen and sustain the assets and resources of a community. For example, one community set up a food cooperative to supply fresh fruit and vegetables at a reasonable cost. In another community, a group of amateur fishermen were helped to set up a fishing group for young people with learning disabilities.

Over to you

Visit the NICE website for the latest guidance on interventions to promote good health and prevent ill health. Are there any interventions that you think might be useful in your area?

Step 4 Plan a public health intervention

A detailed plan will help you to be clear about what you want to achieve, what needs to be done, how it needs to be done, who needs to do it and when it needs to be completed. It will help you to keep track of progress and should describe everything in Table 4.6.

Table 4.6 Use these points to track your progress

Aims	What you are trying to achieve
Objectives	Specific, measurable, achievable, realistic, time-bound
Resources	Finance, time, equipment, skills and venues
Timescales	Milestones for each part of the project
Actions	Who has responsibility for what
Evaluation	How will you know you have been successful? What indicators will you use? What changes do you expect to observe? What will be different? What will be the impact? How can you share what you have done?

Key points | **Top tips**

- Capture what is happening as you go along and record it in as many ways as possible. Try using journals, pictures, photographs, sound and video recordings, and stories. This will help you to bring the HNA alive and make it easier to review your progress in Step 5

Step 5 Conduct a review

HNA is an ongoing process, not a one-off project. The final step is to identify what has been learned by asking these questions:

- What challenges did I overcome?
- What worked really well for the team?
- What else do I need to do?

Also consider how you will update the profile, identify new priorities and maintain the momentum so that HNA becomes an integral part of the way the team works. Then the HNA team can ensure that the services designed and delivered are the most appropriate for the population.

How to avoid the pitfalls of HNAs

Practitioners new to public health often ask how they can avoid the pitfalls of HNA. So here are some top tips from experienced practitioners. Also have a look at Table 4.7.

Key points | **Top tips**

- Be realistic
- Be clear about what you are trying to achieve
- Set clear boundaries, aims and objectives
- Stay focused
- Get others on board and get support
- Take action
- Build on what is already happening
- Set a target date for completion
- Celebrate your success along the way

Table 4.7 HNA pitfalls and how to avoid them

Pitfalls	How to avoid them
Too much information	Focus the HNA on a specific area and have clear aims and objectives
Too little information	Use qualitative and quantitative data. Gather data from a variety of sources
Disagreement among professionals	Set clear agendas and working conditions at the beginning. Appoint a facilitator
Initiatives fall at the first hurdle	Engage the community or target group from the outset
Information but no action	Draw up an action plan and stick to it

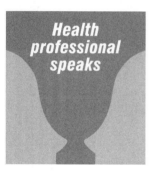

Health professional speaks

Director of public health
Warning! Don't let your health needs assessment be like an elephant with constipation – months of intense straining then a loud report before it all gets dropped.

Over to you

A local housing estate in your area seems to have a significant problem with teenagers misusing alcohol and drugs. Gangs are forming in the park and the elderly residents on the estate are becoming too scared to go to the bowls club in the evenings.

- What types of need are you likely to encounter in this scenario?
- What are your two key objectives?
- Who do you need to involve and why? See Table 4.8.
- What pitfalls are you likely to encounter and how would you overcome them?

Table 4.8 Who to involve and why

Who to involve	Why
Young people	To engage with young people so that you ask the right questions and are sure that the services you develop are suited to their needs
Parents	They are likely to have a useful perspective and additional concerns that you may need to address

School staff	They are vital links with young people and have a wealth of expertise in relating to this age group
School health advisors	They offer close contact with young people in schools as they offer confidential drop-in services
Specialist health promotion staff	To help get the message across about the health issues of drinking and drug misuse
GP and local practice staff	They are likely to have some practice data about the size and nature of the problem
Community drugs team	They have information about what interventions are likely to work and what is already happening
Community adolescent mental health team	They will help you decide the most effective way forward
Police	They will have data about the levels of crime and are likely to have a community presence
Voluntary agencies	Church groups, NSPCC, Barnardo's, etc. may already be offering services
Social services	They will have knowledge and expertise of working with vulnerable young people and communities

There are several ways you could answer these questions and plan this HNA. The types of need you are likely to encounter are poverty, mental health needs, low self-esteem, poor educational attainment, poor housing, inadequate transport and local facilities, and social isolation (elderly population). The key objectives will be to build a picture of the health needs of this population group and to plan an appropriate intervention to meet the identified needs of this population, such as a better drop-in service for primary and secondary students.

Examples of HNAs

Farm Out

The Farm Out project was set up in 2004 to improve the farming community's physical and mental health following an economic crisis in farming. The target population was 700 farms or smallholdings. The participatory HNA used the Dahlgren and Whitehead (1991) framework to guide data collection. The team, led by a public health nurse, gathered information through listening events, focus groups, farm visits, individual interviews, farming events, 248 postal questionnaires and existing community information. The assessment identified the increased risk to farmers and their families of mental health issues, particularly suicide. Strategies were developed to tackle the problem, including a drop-in service at the local agricultural centre, an agricultural chaplain, an outreach mental health worker, a farming life centre, an art project for young farmers and literacy awareness training.

Ribbleton CHT

Ribbleton community health team (CHT) decided to conduct an HNA as the starting point for becoming a practice development unit (CDHPP 2003). The first step was to establish an HNA group from a variety of health professionals, health visitors and district nurses under the leadership of a community development worker. The aim of this group was to profile the population of Ribbleton to identify the priorities and provide a baseline assessment for future developments. They collected data from partner agencies, census data, crime figures, information from schools and data from local GP surgeries.

There was a wealth of information from the public health department, sometimes too much, yet they could find very little on the community itself. The team soon realised that to get a true picture, it would need to engage with the people who lived in the area, and so it set up a series of community focus groups and developed a community questionnaire. The focus groups and the questionnaire revealed that the health need priorities of the community were alcohol and drug misuse, social isolation, youth nuisance, lack of dental care, lack of activities and crime. These priorities were felt across all age groups.

The team then hosted an event to share the findings of the HNA with the whole community and other key stakeholders. Following that event, it was agreed to focus on alcohol and substance misuse as the number one priority. The stakeholder event was a springboard to excellent partnership working, and Ribbleton now has a local action group with its own vision and strategy. The local action group has started to develop interventions to tackle alcohol and substance misuse, such as awareness-raising events and an alcohol education project in primary schools and activity groups. The team are evaluating the impact of the interventions alongside the community.

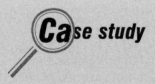

Case study

Homesick mothers

Anne is a midwife working in a small district general hospital in a largely rural area of England. Over the past year, Anne has noticed an influx of Portuguese women arriving for antenatal care and to have their babies. While chatting with some of the women, Anne finds out they have moved to England with their partners to seek work in the agricultural and food industries. They say their accommodation is poor and often temporary. Their incomes are low and there is little public transport in rural areas. Many of them have several very young children and seem unaware of contraceptive services. Some do not speak English and many feel isolated and are missing their homeland.

● Using the five steps, plan an HNA to meet the needs of this group of women and their families.

Conclusion

HNA is the basis of public health practice. This chapter has outlined some of the debate about the nature of need and helped you get to grips with needs assessment and the different perspectives on need. It has taken you through all five steps of the HNA process and offered some frameworks to guide you. Now that you are familiar with the process, you can begin to build a public health approach to your practice and start to use some of your new skills.

RRRRRapid recap

Check your progress so far by working through each of the following questions.

1. What are the four types of need?
2. How does a sociologist's perspective of need differ from an epidemiologist's?
3. What are the key perspectives of HNA?
4. Identify three purposes of HNA.
5. What five steps help to ensure a comprehensive HNA that results in action?

If you have difficulty with more than one of the questions, read through the section again to refresh your understanding before moving on.

References

Acheson, D. (1998) *Independent Inquiry into Inequality in Health: Report*. HMSO, London.

Annett, S. and Rifkin, H. (1996) *Guidelines for Rapid Participatory Appraisal to Assess Community Health Needs*. WHO, Geneva.

Billings, J. (2002) Profiling health needs. In: *Public Health in Policy and Practice* (ed. Cowley, S.). Ballière Tindall, London.

Bowling, A. (2004) *A Review of Quality of Life Measurement Scales*, 3rd edn. Open University Press, Maidenhead, Berks.

Bradshaw, J. (1972) A taxonomy of social need. In: *Problems and Progress in Medical Care*, 6th edn (ed. Maclachlan, G.). Oxford University Press, Oxford.

Bradshaw, J. (1994) The conceptualisation and measurement of need: a social policy perspective. In: *Research the People's Health* (eds. Popay, J. and Edwards, G.). Routledge, London.

Buonfino, A. and Geissendorfer, L. (2006) *Mapping the Unmet Needs of Britain*. www.youngfoundation.org.uk/wp-content/Mapping_Britains_Needs.pdf, accessed 4 January 2007.

Cavanagh, S. and Chadwick, K. (2005) *Health Needs Assessment*. www.nice.org.uk.

CDHPP (2003) *Practice Development Programme*. www.cdhpp.leeds.ac.uk.

Cowley, S. (2000) In: *The Search for Health Needs: Research for Health Visiting Practice* (eds Appleton, J. V. and Cowley, S.). Macmillan, Basingstoke, Hants.

Cowley, S. (2002) *Public Health in Policy and Practice: A Sourcebook for Health Visitors and Community Practitioners*. Ballière Tindall, London.

Dahlgren, G. and Whitehead, M. (1991) *Policies and Strategies to Promote Social Equity in Health*. Institute of Future Studies, Stockholm.

Department of Health (2005) *Creating a Patient-Led NHS*. HMSO, London.

Department of Health (2006) *Our Health, Our Care, Our Say*. HMSO, London.

Health Development Agency (2004) *Health Needs Assessment*. HDA, London.

Hooper, J. and Longworth, P. (2002) *Health Needs Assessment Workbook*. www.hda-online.org.uk/documents/hna.pdf.

Lazenbatt, A. and McMurray, F. (2004) Using participatory rapid appraisal as a tool to assess women's psychosocial health needs in Northern Ireland. *Health Education*, **10**(3), 174–187.

Mitcheson, J. and Cowley, S. (2003) Empowerment or control. An analysis of the extent to which client participation is enabled during the health visitor/client interactions using a structured health needs assessment tool. *International Journal of Nursing Studies*, **40**, 413–426.

Mooney, G. (2003) *Economics, Medicine and Healthcare*, 3rd edn. Prentice Hall, Upper Saddle River NJ.

Murray, S. (1999) Experiences with rapid appraisal in primary care: involving the public in assessing health needs. *British Medical Journal*, **318**, 440–444.

Newdick, C. (2005) *Who Should We Treat? Rights, Rationing and Resources in the NHS*, 2nd edn. Oxford University Press, Oxford.

Orr, J. (1992) Assessing individual and family health needs. In: *Health Visiting: Towards Community Health Nursing* (eds Luker, K. and Orr, J.). Blackwell, Oxford.

Pepall, E., Earnest, J. and James, R. (2007) Understanding community perceptions of health and social needs in a rural Balinese village: results of a rapid participatory appraisal. *Health Promotion International*, **22**, 44–52.

Petersen, D. J. and Alexander, G. R. (2001) *Needs Assessment in Public Health: A Practical Guide for Students and Professionals*. Springer, New York.

Pickin, C. and Leger, S. (1994) *Assessing Health Needs Using the Life Cycle Framework*. Open University Press, Buckingham.

Powell, J. (2003) Cited in Watterson, A. *Public Health in Practice*. Palgrave Macmillan, Basingstoke.

Robinson, J. and Elkan, R. (1996) *Health Needs Assessment: Theory and Practice*. Churchill Livingstone, Edinburgh.

Skinner, S. and Wilson, M. (2005) *Assessing Community Strengths: A Practical Handbook for Planning Capacity Building*. Community Development Foundation, London.

Stanhope, M. and Lancaster, J. (2004) *Community and Public Health Nursing*. Mosby, St Louis MO.

Stevens, A. and Gabby, J. (1991) Needs assessment needs assessment. *Health Trends*, **23**, 20–23.

Wanless, D. (2004) *Securing Good Health for the Whole Population*. HMSO, London.

Yin, R. (1994) *Case Study Research: Design and Methods*, 2nd edn. Sage, Beverly Hills CA.

5
Using evidence in public health practice

Ivy O'Neil

Learning outcomes

By the end of this chapter you should be able to:

★ Identify data useful for health needs assessment

★ Interpret data relevant to your area of public health practice

★ Discuss the advantages and limitations of data

★ Appraise the evidence base for public health interventions and practice

★ Understand the importance of the key concepts of validity and reliability.

Introduction

Public health evidence is widely available. It provides essential information for understanding and assessing the health needs of a community in order to plan health service provision to improve the health of the public. It helps you to:

● predict and study the trends and changing pattern of health and illness

● make decisions on preventive intervention strategies

● evaluate the effectiveness and efficiency of public health-care strategies and interventions.

This chapter is about how practitioners can use and interpret evidence. It explains how practitioners can obtain the best evidence to support their practice and how to make public health evidence meaningful and applicable to practice. The first part explores epidemiological evidence, or data, where to find it, how to interpret it and the advantages and limitations of using it to identify health and social needs of your community. The second part considers the knowledge and skills to appraise evidence when selecting an intervention to address the health needs you have identified.

Epidemiology is a key part of public health practice. The central paradigm of epidemiology is that disease patterns in populations can be analysed systematically. The basic principle of epidemiology is that diseases occur in patterns in the community and that these patterns are predictable. Epidemiology is a science of relating disease patterns to population groups, even if the starting point is the impact of disease on individuals. Epidemiology helps to establish health strategies that implement national priorities and meet local health needs.

Epidemiology also helps to monitor and evaluate changes in health and illness and the delivery of health services.

Epidemiological data is collected using an epidemiological approach. It is commonly used to measure health and produces quantitative data. It is largely based on the assumption that expert knowledge of ill health is the primary descriptor of health. It is a medical approach to measuring health. More recently, epidemiological data has expanded to include qualitative data about people's experience of health and illness, but there is less of this data and people argue about its value. We will return to this subject later in the chapter.

Evidence base

Read Moon, G. and Gould, M. (2001) *Epidemiology: An Introduction*. Open University Press, Buckingham.

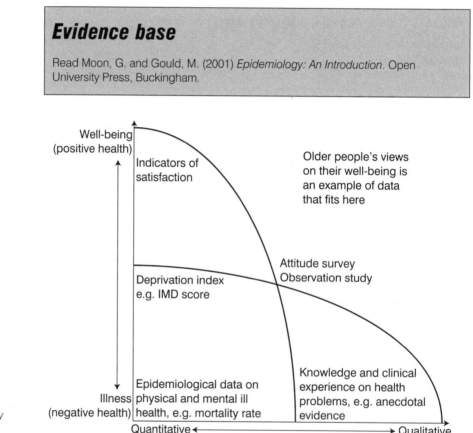

Figure 5.1 A modified version of Stacey's agreement and certainty matrix

Figure 5.1 shows that much available knowledge is quantitative data (in the bottom left-hand corner). It consists of data that is largely defined by professionals. For example, there is much more empirical data about coronary heart disease (CHD) than about older people's own definitions of well-being. To get a full picture of health or illness, empirical data about CHD has to be interpreted in a wider public health context. Figure 5.1 is adapted from Stacey's agreement and certainty matrix (Stacey 1999); it shows the types of evidence that relate to health and illness.

Useful data

Quantitative data and qualitative data are the two main types of epidemiological data available to the public health practitioner (Table 5.1). You will probably need both types of data to make an accurate assessment of health needs. The type of data, its complexity and its comprehensiveness will depend on the objectives of your health needs assessment (HNA). The very first question you need to ask is, what is the purpose of this HNA?

Table 5.1 Sources of qualitative and quantitative data

Quantitative data	Qualitative data
Quantitative research findings	Qualitative research findings
Mortality, morbidity, prevalence, incidence	Knowledge of practitioners and people who work with your target population
Data on hospital admissions, discharges, operations and waiting lists	Knowledge in the community and views of people in the community
GP practice data on the health of the practice population	Knowledge of the community
Public health reports and national statistics	
Public Health Observatory	
Services available and initiatives implemented	

Quantitative data

Quantitative data is collected through a deductive approach using a body of knowledge on the subject. It is often about numerical analysis. The data can be factual information (age) or research-generated classifications (e.g. very satisfied, very dissatisfied). Results are usually population descriptors rather than subtle and in-depth findings of individual behaviour. Quantitative data can be descriptive or can be used to answer a very specific question by collating measurable data to test whether or not the answer is true. Representative data can be produced to describe a whole population, often in quite minute detail. Findings are analysed using statistical packages such as **SPSS**. Tables and graphs can be produced to work out the relationship between sets of data. Quantitative data is obtained using research methods such as questionnaires to gain measurable information. It provides the evidence for evidence-based medicine.

Quantitative data from epidemiological studies is readily available from national reports released by the Department of Health and the Office for National Statistics as well as other published research. Local data is available from the Public Health Observatory, Public Health Reports (PHR), primary care trusts (PCTs) and hospital admission and discharge data. Practitioners may have their own statistics such as

⚷ Keywords

SPSS
Statistical Package for Social Sciences: this is computer software that helps to analyse complex quantitative data

profiles of a specific group of patients or clients. For example, a midwife or health visitor is likely to have data on the number of breastfeeding mothers, whereas a nurse in outpatients may know the number of Asian men with diabetes who visit the diabetic services. The list is endless.

Table 5.2 Useful terms and their meanings

Term	Meaning
Prevalence	All the people in a population with the condition at a given point in time or over a given period of time. Usually expressed as a number of people with the condition per 1,000 in the total population
Point prevalence	The proportion of people in a population with a condition at one point in time
Period prevalence	The proportion of people in a population that had a condition during a specific time period
Incidence	Refers to new cases of a condition that develop in a population over a specific period of time; usually expressed as number of new cases per 1,000
Morbidity	The state of being disease (e.g. cancer registration; notification of congenital abnormalities; notification of infectious disease)
Mortality – dying	Mortality rate for a specific disease is the risk of dying from that cause; usually expressed as the number of deaths per 1,000 per year
Crude mortality rate	Number of deaths per 1,000 population per year
Age- and category- specific mortality rate	Mortality rate for a specific age group and a specific category such as male and female, or specific cause of death such as lung cancer
Standardised mortality rate	Mortality takes into account the fact that some causes of death are more common at different ages and so the rates are adjusted for the specific age bands
Standardised mortality ratio (SMR)	This compares the actual number of events in an area with the expected number of events based on mortality rates of a reference population (e.g. England and Wales). The SMR is a ratio of observed to expected number of deaths

Evidence base

Here are some websites where you can find useful quantitative epidemiological data:

- the Office for National Statistics – click in the 'Browse by theme' box and select 'Health Search' for the statistics that interest you
- Neighbourhood Statistics – type in the postcode or the area that interests you
- the Association of Public Health Observatories (APHO)

Qualitative data

Qualitative epidemiological data is often, somewhat disparagingly, known as popular or lay epidemiology (Moon and Gould 2001). It refers to the views, opinions and knowledge of ordinary people and it can help to give a more in-depth understanding of people's own views or it can sometimes clarify the key issues. Most illness never comes to the attention of health-care professionals; it is dealt with by over-the-counter medicines and other remedies, or perhaps it goes ignored and undiagnosed, part of the 'health iceberg'. In that sense, lay epidemiological data offers an important insight into how disease is commonly understood and treated. Moreover, the patient or client perspective is increasingly recognised as crucially important, not only to identify needs and develop appropriate services but also to assess the impact of services.

Qualitative data is collected through an inductive approach to gain insight into people's lives. Public health practitioners search for in-depth information that could help explain the issues as well as data on attitudes, values and judgements. Then they try to identify common themes from the data by looking for similarities and differences of perspective. Here are some ways to collect qualitative data:

- interviews
- patient or client stories
- focus group discussions
- observations
- video evidence
- diaries.

Qualitative data can be used to address a variety of different questions:

- It helps to reveal what health or well-being means in people's lives. An open-ended discussion with a few people could begin to tease out the issues.
- It helps to explain how different individuals and groups behave and interact. For example, what do young people say about sexual health and how do they actually behave in practice? This might involve a mixture of unstructured interviews, observation of participants, and field notes on what happens on a night out.
- It helps to classify different types of behaviour. Why do some people act on health messages whereas others don't?

Evidence base

Read Wilcock, P. M., Brown, G. C., Bateson, J., Carver, J. and Machin, S. (2003) Using patient stories to inspire quality improvement within the NHS Modernisation Agency collaborative programmes. *Journal of Clinical Nursing*, **12**(3), 422–430. This will help you understand the importance of patient and client narratives in needs assessment, service design and service delivery.

One of the reasons qualitative data attracts criticism is that it is seen by some as unscientific. It can be difficult to reproduce and the data analysis depends on the researcher's interpretation. It does not give a scientific, factual measure of illness or health. Strictly speaking, qualitative data can only help to provide data about perspectives of what *might* be. The purpose is to produce rich data about experiences, but a sample of five or six cases will never be truly representative of a whole population. Do not overstate your qualitative data. But equally, do not overstate your quantitative data. Just because something can be measured, the measurements aren't necessarily an accurate description of people's lives. For example, people with disabilities have said that quantitative data comes from measuring what they can or cannot do, but the main barrier they face is other people's attitudes not the bits of their bodies that don't work. Measurements of a disabled person's functionality might imply that they can't do certain things. Measurements of other people's attitudes or the disabling environment might imply that things in society need to change.

Another contentious issue is the scientific outsider. Scientists say that valid knowledge can only be gleaned by objective, dispassionate observation with findings that can be replicated in any setting by anyone. Therefore any data that is collected in any other way is seen as anecdotal, uninformed and even dangerous (Moon and Gould 2001). But other people see experts such as doctors and epidemiologists as removed from the frame of analysis and focused only on what causes disease. There is a tendency to assume that the results of epidemiological data generated in this way apply uniformly and equally to everyone. But they don't. Many of us know someone who smoked 40 cigarettes a day and lived to be 93. Consequently, many people are not persuaded by the evidence and argue that the most reliable data comes from insider views. The key message is that public health practitioners have to be flexible in ways of knowing and use both types of data to get a picture of a community's health needs.

Population data

Population data helps practitioners to identify public health issues. Similar to disease patterns and disease frequencies, population characteristics change over time and they differ from group to group and from place to place. The increase or decrease of illnesses and the change in pattern of health and illness could be due to a change in population characteristics. For example, an increase in type 2 diabetes in a particular area could be due to an increase in the number of people from South Asia, or a high number of teenage pregnancies in an area could be explained by its high number of young people. Population data enables public health practitioners to describe the size and key characteristics of a population. Together with morbidity, mortality and socio-economic status, it can build pictures and patterns of a community's health. Box 5.1 shows some common ways to express population data.

Box 5.1

How to calculate mortality and morbidity rates

$$\text{Rate} = \frac{\text{numerator}}{\text{denominator}}$$

$$\text{Mortality rate} = \frac{\text{number of people that have died}}{\text{total population}}$$

$$\text{Morbidity rate} = \frac{\text{number of people that have an illness}}{\text{total population}}$$

The rate is often expressed as the number of cases per 1,000 or 100,000 population, or it can be given as a percentage

Mortality and morbidity data

A population's health is most commonly described by mortality and morbidity data. The mortality rate is a measure of the death rate. When a person dies, someone who can verify the age, sex, occupation and usual address of the dead person must register the death. A medical practitioner or coroner has to identify the underlying cause of death. The registrar has to send this information to the Office for National Statistics, where the cause of death is coded using the international classification of disease (ICD; WHO 1998).

Mortality rates appear very factual and scientific as they are derived from counting numbers of deaths from classified illnesses. However, they measure ill health and reflect a medical model of health. The accuracy of information depends on what is written on the death certificate and how the information was classified. A decrease in mortality rate does not always mean the population is healthier. Decreased mortality rates may mean an increase in chronic ill health, more seriously disabled people and more long-term conditions. It could demonstrate that more people survive because of improvements in health care and advanced technology but they survive in a debilitated condition.

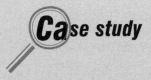
Case study

Mr Jones is run over

Mr Jones, aged 59, suffered from early symptoms of Alzheimer's disease. He was run over by a car when he wandered into a busy road. Dr Smith was called to the scene and recorded the cause of death as a road traffic accident. Her colleague, Dr White, thought that Mr Jones's cause of death may have been Alzheimer's disease.

- With your colleagues, discuss how Dr Smith would know the mental state of the person at the time of the accident.
- With your colleagues, discuss the traffic conditions and the circumstances of the driver at the time.
- With your colleagues, discuss how Dr Smith and Dr White would determine the actual cause of death.

Crude mortality rates can be a very misleading way of comparing the mortality in different populations. The single most important determinant of mortality is age. Populations can vary significantly in their age structures and this also has to be considered. Age-adjusted or standardised mortality rates are a more useful measure. The standardised mortality ratio (SMR) can be used to compare death rates between two or more populations and control for age structure. If the SMR is 100 then the standard population and the population studied have the same mortality rate. If the SMR is greater than 100 then the mortality rate is higher in the population studied; if the SMR is less than 100 then the mortality rate is lower in the population studied. For example, if your working area has an SMR of 114 then you will know that the mortality rate is 14 per cent higher than the mortality rate in England and Wales.

$$\text{SMR} = \frac{\text{observed number of deaths}}{\text{expected number of deaths}}$$

Morbidity data is mainly generated from health service activity. It provides information on patterns and variations in health and ill health and is more useful when analysing trends and causes of ill health. It is collated from infectious disease notification, cancer registration, and hospital and primary care activity. Box 5.2 shows how to calculate the two important measures that are used.

There are some difficulties in using morbidity data. Morbidity data depends on patients or clients presenting to a health-care practitioner and recognising that they are ill. But some people do not go to a health-care practitioner; they may live with their pain or seek alternative sources of help. Cultural and personal beliefs influence what people do when they have a pain. Another source of problems is the way that diseases are diagnosed and classified. Finally, there is a general lack of data about some specific conditions that are not categorised separately; an example is post-natal depression.

Box 5.2

How to calculate incidence and prevalence

$$\text{Prevalence} = \frac{\text{number of persons ill at a specific time}}{\text{total number in the group at a specific time}}$$

$$\text{Incidence} = \frac{\text{number of new cases}}{\text{total population at risk}}$$

The population at risk is all the people who could potentially become a new case

Census data

A census is a survey of all people and households in the country. Every 10 years in England and Wales the country is divided into enumeration districts and every householder is legally obliged to complete a census

Keywords

Demographic data

Demographic data shows the characteristics of the population in a particular area such as age, gender, socio-economic variables and level of deprivation. Demography is the study of human populations, their size, distribution and transitions

Socio-economic data

Socio-economic data describes aspects of people's lives, such as income, employment, class and level of education. It can be seen as a more holistic way of understanding health. It involves looking at the different social and economic factors influencing health (Dahlgren and Whitehead 1991) and produces a social model of health. The economic and sociological aspects of health have long been acknowledged (Acheson 1998; Black *et al.* 1980). These aspects can describe a wider definition of health and well-being and can be used to describe or even explain different aspects of illness. Socio-economic data can be used to describe ill health and wider aspects of health inequalities and deprivation

questionnaire. It is the most complete source of information about the population. It provides information, key **demographic data**, such as age and sex, and **socio-economic data** relating to occupation, accommodation and amenities. The most recent census was in April 2001. Census data is available at different levels, such as health authority, district and ward. Using census data it is possible to describe the demography of an area or to analyse the association between health and socio-economic variables such as housing and unemployment. Since 1991 the census has also included this question: Does the person have a long-term illness or disability that limits their activities and ability to work? This gives data on self-reported long-term limiting illness.

Evidence base

Find census data at the Office for National Statistics website

Census data provides extremely useful information for HNA; it is considered largely accurate and complete. But a big census creates its own difficulties and the data should be used with caution as it quickly becomes out of date and may be affected by issues at the time of the survey. For example, it was estimated that there were 1 million people 'missing' from the 1991 census predominantly from the young male population, aged 19–30. It has been suggested that missing people wanted to avoid poll tax payments. If a public health practitioner relied solely on this information to assess the needs of this group, then their assessment would probably be flawed.

Over to you

Can you see any weaknesses in the census questions in Table 5.3? Think about these two points and discuss them with your colleagues:

- There are many different countries and cultures in Africa and Asia, yet the tendency is to put lots of other countries together as a similar group.
- What does this mean for the provision of services?

Table 5.3 Data collection by ethnic group

1991 Census question	2001 Census question
White	White – British White – Irish White – Any other White background (please write in)
(Others …)	Mixed – White/Black Caribbean Mixed – White/Black African Mixed – White/Asian Any other mixed background (please write in)

Table 5.3 Data collection by ethnic group (continued)

1991 Census question	2001 Census question
Black Caribbean	Black or Black British: Caribbean
Black African	Black or Black British: African
Black others (please describe)	Black or Black British Any other background (please write in)
Indian	Asian or Asian British Indian
Pakistani	Asian or Asian British Pakistani
Bangladeshi	Asian or Asian British Bangladeshi
Asian – other (please describe)	Asian or Asian British Any other background (please write in)
Chinese	Chinese or other ethnic group
Any other ethnic group (please describe)	Any other (please write in)

Measures of deprivation

In 2000 the index of multiple deprivations (IMD 2000) replaced the Jarman score (Jarman 1984) as the method for measuring deprivation in geographical localities. The IMD is used by the Department of Communities and Local Government (DCLG) to measure deprivation across 36 social and economic indicators. The index of deprivation (ID 2004) uses more recent data and contains seven domains: income deprivation; employment deprivation; health deprivation and disability; education, skills and training deprivation; barriers to housing and services; living environment deprivation; and crime. It measures deprivation in a small area. People may be counted in one or more of the domains, depending on the number of types of deprivation they experience. The overall IMD is conceptualised as a weighted area-level aggregation of these specific dimensions of deprivation (Office of the Deputy Prime Minister 2004). Although this information is very useful for indicating levels of deprivation and for attracting additional resources, relative deprivation doesn't help to plan services.

Over to you

Look at the most recent profile of your area. Use the Public Health Observatory or Neighbourhood Statistics to locate the health profile of the area that interests you. Consider these questions:

- Is the area you have chosen an affluent area or a highly deprived area?
- Would the health summary apply in the same way to all areas in the same region?
- What about the population? Is there a high concentration of young families or older people?
- What about the knowledge of your colleagues? What is the experience of the people you work with or have contact with? How does their knowledge compare with the figures in the profile?
- What would your patients or clients think? Would they recognise the issues you present to them or would they have a different view?

Appraising public health data

Public health data is obtained from various processes and you will need to assess the data for accuracy, completeness, timeliness and validity (Carr *et al.* 2007):

- **Accuracy** – how has the data been collected and interpreted? Even objective data can receive several interpretations. The accuracy of data depends very much on the processes adopted.
- **Completeness** – does the data include everyone who should have been included?
- **Timeliness** – how recent is the data? Data on age and sex may still be relevant two years after collection, but data about outbreaks of food poisoning may not.
- **Validity** – is the data appropriate for what you wish to find out?

Over to you

Data can be misleading. Make a list of the reasons why. Think about some of the data that you now rely on or used to rely on. Do you have any questions about these aspects of the data?

- Errors or bias in data collection
- Interpretation of the data
- Coding systems in computerised records
- Accessibility of health care
- Different clinical practice in different places

Key points Top tips

- There are very complex interactions between the risk factors for a disease, such as economic, social and environmental factors. There are many challenges in using epidemiological data
- Over-reliance on epidemiological data that is purely quantitative and focused on disease may distract us from the underlying causes of ill health
- Inaccurate data can give an incomplete and wrong impression of a population's health
- Epidemiological data suggests a relationship between cause and effects rather than proof from the facts that certain conditions will cause illness, such as smoking causes lung cancer (Parascandola 1998)

HNA is not a complicated process, but complexity arises because there are no universal definitions of 'health' and 'needs' (Chapter 4). The validity of the data depends on your personal view about health and needs. Data that is meaningful to you may not be meaningful to other people if they define health in a different way or if they use a different parameter to decide which needs count as unmet needs. Data and data collection create many challenges. Interpreting and presenting public health data can be a highly political activity. People often present data to justify funding and many people think that the purpose of HNA is the justification of funding. Table 5.4 lists some questions to ask when you handle public health data.

Table 5.4 Questions to ask when handling public health data

Aspect	Questions to ask
Data	How accurate is the data? Is it complete, timely and valid? What coding system is used? Is it computerised? Can you identify the recording method used?
Method	Is the method of data collection appropriate? What is the potential for bias? Sampling technique – is it representative of the population? Questionnaire design – what questions were asked and how were they asked? Interviews – is the schedule well designed and the interviewer trained in this type of data collection?
Analysis	Was the correct method used to analyse the data? How is the data cross-referenced with other forms of data?
Report	Is the report balanced and fair or does it manipulate the data in favour of specific points or issues?
General	Have the correct procedure and guidelines been followed, e.g. confidentiality? Has the information been compromised to meet a different target or agenda?

Interpreting public health data

Keywords

Evidence-based practice

The phrase 'evidence-based' implies the concept of scientific rationality; the word 'practice' refers to individual practitioner behaviour (Lockett 1997)

Once you have gathered and appraised your data, consider which interventions you need. Most published public health data has already been analysed by researchers and will be interpreted for you. As a practitioner, it is more important that you know how to interpret the available data to make it meaningful to you, so you can use it in your **evidence-based practice**.

Epidemiological data is usually quantitative. It is a useful way to give a numerical picture of a population's health, be it good or bad. You can easily see the trends for some conditions. But to get a fuller picture of a community's health, you need to combine epidemiological data with demographic data, including socio-economic status. When resources are limited, it is acceptable to interpret the epidemiological data with the demographic data and set your priorities for service planning.

In recent years, more importance has been placed on listening to local voices plus public and user involvement. *A Stronger Local Voice* (Department of Health 2006) sets out the government's plans for the future of patient and public involvement in health and social care. One aspect of these plans is to establish a link between local involvement networks, existing voluntary and community organisations, and interested individuals to promote public and community influence in health and social care.

Over to you

Here are some points from the Acheson Report (Acheson 1998):

- Mortality rates for cerebral vascular disease are significantly higher for all migrant groups except those born in East Africa.
- Mortality rates for lung cancer are lower in people born in the Caribbean, Asia and Africa, and higher in people born in Scotland and Ireland.
- South Asians have a tendency to central obesity and insulin resistance, which predisposes them to diabetes and coronary heart disease.
- Tuberculosis is more common in Pakistanis, Bangladeshis and Black Africans.
- Alcohol consumption is lower in ethnic minority groups and there is total abstinence among Muslim groups.

Search out the national statistics or regional statistics for coronary heart disease, tuberculosis and lung cancer. Then look at a local public health reports; you can find them from the local public health website or PCT website. Now look at the demographic structure of the population in your area, including age, gender, ethnic group and religion. Also find out the IMD score of your area; IMD scores are given in the 2001 census data. Discuss your findings with your colleagues.

- Would they agree with you?
- What do their experiences tell you?
- What would their record tell you?
- If you asked your clients, would they tell you the same thing?
- What do you think about the validity and the reliability of all the information?
- How can you make sense of it?

To create a patient-led NHS (Department of Health 2005), the government wants to change the whole system so there is more choice, more personalised care and real empowerment of people to improve their health, and it wants to move from a service-led NHS to a patient-led NHS, where the service works with patients or clients to support them with their health needs.

If the information is not accurately interpreted, any strategies to improve health will not be well grounded. You need to consider many variables when you interpret public health data, as you can see from the above exercise, and you need to consider all the other information. Other practitioners in your area may have relevant and valid information that could make your interpretation richer and more comprehensive. The patients or clients in your area may also tell you a different story than is in the public health report. To make the public health data meaningful, take a broader view of the available information so that you get a full picture of people's health. Otherwise the service provision will not be appropriate and you may wonder why there is a low uptake of your excellent service, which you carefully and painstakingly designed.

Confidentiality

Confidentiality is a key issue when reporting HNAs and public health data, particularly qualitative data. Take care to protect the public and treat all health data with the strictest confidentiality. Information governance is a framework for handling information in a confidential and secure manner appropriate to ethical and quality standards. It covers the Caldicott recommendations on the use of patient-identifiable information (Department of Health 1997) and the Freedom of Information Act 2000. Many of the issues you investigate will probably be sensitive and will need to be handled accordingly when you make HNA reports.

Working with evidence

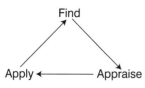

Figure 5.2 Stages of evidence-based practice

Having used public health data to identify the health needs of your community, the next step is to decide what interventions are most appropriate. In other words, decide what evidence you should use as a basis for your practice. Evidence-based practice is a process of finding, appraising and applying the evidence (Figure 5.2). Its ultimate goal is to support practitioners in their decision making in order to eliminate practices that are ineffective, inappropriate, too expensive and potentially dangerous (Hamer and Collinson 2005).

Find the evidence

Figure 5.3 shows the different forms of evidence as a continuum. However, within a positivist approach, not all evidence has equal status. Positivism would see the randomised control trial as the gold standard for evidence. Few researchers would believe in a totally posivitist approach; most would see a need for a variety of sources of evidence to give a broad range of perspectives.

Exploratory   **Positivist**

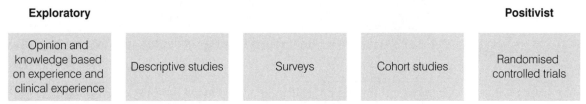

| Opinion and knowledge based on experience and clinical experience | Descriptive studies | Surveys | Cohort studies | Randomised controlled trials |

Figure 5.3 Continuum of evidence

A literature review is the first step when a public health practitioner embarks on a new initiative. Literature reviews can be done in many ways and you will probably be familiar them. There are a huge number of journals in hundreds of databases – 20,000 medical journals alone – and this can be overwhelming to the busy health-care worker. *Evidence-Based Healthcare and Public Health*, published by Elsevier (see the website of Harcourt International), provides abstracts of relevant studies and may be a good starting point. Another possible starting point is the website of the National Library for Public Health.

The UK Cochrane Centre and the NHS Centre for Reviews and Dissemination at the University of York are funded by the Department of Health to provide reviews on the effectiveness of health-care interventions. The search results are limited to reports where the research methods are seen as producing scientifically valid findings. Many research bodies produce accessible summaries of key findings from a project or a whole research programme. One of the best examples of these bodies is the Joseph Rowntree Foundation.

Evidence base

Go to the websites of the UK Cochrane Centre, the University of York and the Joseph Rowntree Foundation to read reviews of research findings.

Evidence can enhance clinical judgement about what interventions are most suitable but it cannot replace clinical judgement. There may be times when the evidence is not sufficiently robust but to do nothing is not an option.

Reflective activity

Can you recall a situation in the past when you have not been able to find sufficient evidence to support an intervention? What did you do and what were the consequences?

Evidence base

Read Humpris, D. (2005) Types of evidence. In: *Achieving Evidence-Based Practice: A Handbook for Practitioners*, 2nd edn (eds Hamer, S. and Collinson, G.). Ballière Tindall, Edinburgh.

Appraise the evidence

To judge the quality and applicability of research evidence about interventions, appraise the published literature in much the same way as you appraise the public health data. Here are some questions to ask:

- Was the research design appropriate?
- Was the method rigorous?
- Was the analysis valid?
- How can you apply the results to your setting?

This chapter does not give detailed formats for appraising every type of research evidence. The Critical Appraisal Skills Programme (CASP), available from the Public Health Resource Unit (PHRU), will help you develop skills to find and make sense of research evidence and put it into practice.

Over to you

From your literature searches, identify a piece of research that you wish to appraise. What method was used to collect the data? Go to the PHRU website, download the appropriate critical appraisal tool and use it to do an appraisal.

Validity and reliability

Validity and reliability are key ideas in evidence appraisal. Validity is about whether the evidence is accepted or approved as the truth. Reliability is about whether the evidence is accurate and representative and whether it can be replicated. Valid methods are methods that are appropriate for measuring what the researchers set out to measure (Bowling 2005). Does a given indicator measure the underlying attribute? Reliable results are results that can be replicated in the population you intend to study. If you are appraising a quantitative study, was the sample size appropriate for its population size and will it be appropriate for your population size? If you are appraising a qualitative study, did it include enough people to cover the range of issues that could emerge? How were the cases selected? Did the sampling strategy contain any biases?

Evidence base

Go to the Health Knowledge website and read *Interpretation of Published Research Articles: Critical Appraisal* by K. Enock.

Key points | **Top tips**

- Look critically at summaries of research findings and question the evidence
- Are the researchers telling you what they have found out or are they giving their recommendations under the guise of research?
- Have the researchers told you the basis for their analysis? Have they explained their methods and sampling techniques?
- Did the researchers adopt a reasonable approach?

Apply the evidence

To use evidence confidently, you need to be able to judge its rigour and its applicability to your practice (Humpris 2005). You also need good knowledge and understanding of your work context:

> Evidence derived from scientific studies is important, for an intervention to be successful, it requires an understanding of local contexts and circumstances of local professionals' knowledge bases, commitment and engagement and detailed assessment of the particular population at whom the intervention is aimed.

> Kelly *et al.* (2004)

This brings us full circle. To apply evidence, you will need to evaluate your interventions and this will generate more evidence for you and other practitioners.

Conclusion

HNA is at the heart of public health practice. You must be able to interpret public health evidence to assess the health of a population and make informed decisions about your health interventions. There are vast amounts of data, so you will need to find the most useful items to give you a true picture of your population's health. Health is multidimensional and influenced by many factors (Dahlgren and Whitehead 1991). To make sense of a community's health needs, you will need a wide range of information and a good understanding of the concepts of health and need.

Effective interventions are based on correct information about a population. You need to consider many variables when you interpret public health data. Quantitative data can demonstrate the health of a population and illustrate trends in health and ill health. Demographic data shows the characteristics of the population in your area. Socio-economic data can reveal the financial and human resources of an area. Qualitative data can help to uncover the 'real' needs of the people you serve. Central to this analysis are engaging the public and empowering the people who use your service; engagement and empowerment are important in influencing the policies that improve health and health-care provision (Warburton 2006).

When you have a comprehensive picture of the community, you can determine the appropriate intervention to meet the community's needs. Find, appraise and apply the evidence about the appropriate intervention, then you will be ready to implement and evaluate that intervention.

𝘙𝘙𝘙𝘙*Rapid recap*

Check your progress so far by working through each of the following questions.

1. Name the data you would use to measure health.
2. What can demographic data tell you?
3. What four factors should you consider when appraising data?
4. What tool is needed to appraise the evidence for public health interventions?
5. What is the difference between validity and reliability?

If you have difficulty with more than one of the questions, read through the section again to refresh your understanding before moving on.

References

Acheson, D. (1998) *Independent Inquiry into Inequality in Health: Report*. HMSO, London.

Black, D., Morris, J., Smith, C. and Townsend, P. (1980) *Inequalities in Health: Report of a Working Party*. Department of Health and Social Security, London.

Bowling, A. (2005) *Measuring Health. A Review of Quality of Life Measurement Scales*, 3rd edn. Open University Press, Maidenhead, Berks.

Carr, S., Unwin, N. and Pless-Mulloli, T. (2007) *An Introduction to Public Health and Epidemiology*. Open University Press, Maidenhead, Berks.

Dahlgren, G. and Whitehead, M. (1991) *Policies and Strategies to Promote Social Equity in Health*. Institute of Future Studies, Stockholm.

Department of Health (1997) *Report on the Review of Patient-Identifiable Information*. HMSO, London.

Department of Health (2005) *Creating a Patient-led NHS*. HMSO, London.

Department of Health (2006) *A Stronger Local Voice*. HMSO, London.

Hamer, S. and Collinson, G. (2005) *Achieving Evidence-Based Practice: A Handbook for Practitioners*, 2nd edn. Ballière Tindall, Edinburgh.

Humpris, D. (2005) Types of evidence. In: *Achieving Evidence-Based Practice: A Handbook for Practitioners*, 2nd edn (eds Hamer, S. and Collinson, G.). Ballière Tindall, Edinburgh.

ID (2004) *The English Indices of Deprivation 2004*. Neighbourhood Renewal Unit, Office of the Deputy Prime Minister, London.

IMD (2000) *Measuring Multiple Deprivation at the Small Area Level: The Indices of Deprivation 2000*. DETR, London.

Jarman, B. (1984) Underprivileged areas: validation and distribution of scores. *British Medical Journal*, **289**, 1587–1592.

Kelly, M. P., Speller, V. and Meyrick, J. (2004) *Getting Evidence Into Practice in Public Health*. Health Development Agency, London.

Lockett, T. (1997) Traces of evidence. *Healthcare Today*, July/August, p. 16.

Moon, G. and Gould, M. (2001) *Epidemiology: An Introduction*. Open University Press, Buckingham.

Office of the Deputy Prime Minister (2004) *The English Indices of Deprivation 2004*. Revised summary. ODPM, London.

Parascandola, M. (1998) Epidemiology: second-rate science. *Public Health Reports*, **113**(4), 312–320.

Stacey, R. D. (1999) *Strategic Management and Organisational Dynamics: The Challenge of Complexity*. Financial Times/Prentice Hall, New York.

Warburton, D. (2006) *Evaluation of Your Health: Your Care Your Say*. Department of Health, London.

Wilcock, P. M., Brown, G. C., Bateson, J., Carver, J. and Machin, S. (2003) Using patient stories to inspire quality improvement within the NHS Modernisation Agency collaborative programmes. *Journal of Clinical Nursing*, **12**(3), 422–430.

World Health Organization (1998) *International Classification of Diseases*, 10th revn. WHO, Geneva.

6
Public health interventions

Jane Goodman-Brown and Mary Gottwald

Learning outcomes

By the end of this chapter you should be able to:

★ Define health promotion

★ Understand the different approaches to health promotion

★ Select the most appropriate interventions to meet the identified needs of the individual or population

★ Apply one of the models of health promotion to your own practice.

Introduction

Health for all (HFA) has been on the World Health Organization's agenda since the Alma-Ata Declaration of 1978 and is now seen as a challenge for the twenty-first century (Katz *et al*. 2002). The UK government has published policies to facilitate HFA (Chapter 1): *Saving Lives: Our Healthier Nation* (Department of Health 1999), the NHS plan (Department of Health 2000) and National Service Frameworks (NSFs) for mental health, coronary heart disease, older people, children, long-term conditions and the forthcoming NSF on chronic obstructive pulmonary disease. *Choosing Health* (Department of Health 2004) says that health promotion is central to the NHS and is therefore important to all health and social care professionals. This chapter explores health promotion and considers the most appropriate and effective interventions for improving health and responding to need.

Definitions of health promotion

It is some years since the World Health Organization (WHO) became an advocate of health promotion (Thibeault and Hebert 1997), partly because it recognised the increase in medical costs and loss of productivity due to unhealthy behaviours (Anderson *et al*. 1999; Thibeault and Hebert 1997). Here are some definitions of health promotion:

> The process of enabling people to increase control over and improve their health. To reach a state of complete physical, mental and social well being an individual or group must be able to identify and realise aspirations to satisfy needs and to change and cope with the environment.

> WHO (1986)

Health promotion is about keeping healthy, living a healthy lifestyle, preventing illness, and preventing any existing illness from becoming worse.

Patient UK (2007)

Behaviour motivated by the desire to increase well-being and actualize human health potential.

Pender *et al.* (2006, p. 7)

The first and third definitions focus on empowering and enabling people to help them decide that they will change their unhealthy behaviours.

Reflective activity

Think about the three definitions. What do they have in common? What is the key point for you to consider?

One of the aims of the White Paper *Choosing Health* (Department of Health 2004) is to enable people to choose healthier lifestyles and to have greater control over their health. There are clear links between this White Paper and the definitions above.

The terms 'health promotion' and 'health education' are sometimes used interchangeably and this causes confusion. Health education is one aspect of health promotion; it tends to focus on one person at a time and gives them information on how they can improve their health and start to change their behaviour (Ewles and Simnett 2003). Health promotion is a wider concept that covers a range of activities:

- Preventive health services include screening and immunisation programmes.
- Community work helps communities identify and address their health concerns. An example is working with a group of mothers to address their health priorities.
- Organisational development helps organisations such as the NHS develop the health of their staff, perhaps by offering healthy choices in the canteens or by providing exercise facilities.
- Healthy public policy means that the healthy choice is the easy choice. Practitioners lobby politicians to formulate healthy public policy (Milio 1986).
- Environmental health measures improve the environment so it is conducive to health, including air pollution and noise pollution. An example is the smoking ban in public places introduced in England on 1 July 2007. Wales, Ireland and Scotland had already introduced similar bans (Ewles and Simnett 2003).

Levels of health promotion

Health promotion can be done at three levels – primary, secondary and tertiary – so that nurses and other health-care practitioners consider how to treat people who are ill but also how to maintain the health of people who are well (Sidell *et al.* 2003):

- **Primary** – healthy people are empowered to follow a healthy lifestyle and to use preventive services such as immunisation, so that new cases of disease are prevented. Examples are a campaign on healthy eating aimed at parents to prevent obesity in children or a programme aimed at raising children's awareness about the hazards of smoking so they do not start to smoke.

- **Secondary** – people who have an illness or disease are helped to recognise the impact of unhealthy behaviours on signs and symptoms of their condition and encouraged to seek early treatment as this will reduce the harm they suffer. An example is a programme that helps a person with diabetes to maintain a healthy diet. Secondary health promotion may also encourage people to use screening procedures to detect, diagnose and treat disease as early as possible.

- **Tertiary** – people with a long-term condition are encouraged to participate in rehabilitation and to change their lifestyle to reduce complications and promote functional independence. An example is a cardiac rehabilitation programme (Godfrey 2003).

Reflective activity

Think of situations in your workplace where you have come across the three levels of health promotion. What were the activities in these situations?

The three levels of health promotion emphasise the applicability of health promotion theory and practice to the whole population.

Approaches to health promotion

Table 6.1 shows some approaches to health promotion. Your choice of approach will depend on the needs assessment, your aims and values, and your preferred way of working. Ewles and Simnett (2003) suggest that choice of approach also depends on whether the aim is to comply with a programme or to enable informed choice by a patient or client. It is essential that you understand the different approaches and the assumptions behind them.

Table 6.1 Approaches to health promotion

Approach	Aim	How the aim is achieved
Medical approach	Freedom from medically defined disease	Medical intervention, such as contraceptive services
Behaviour change approach	Clients change their behaviour to limit their health risks	Persuasive education to alter behaviour, such as teaching clients how to eat a healthy diet
Educational approach	Clients get the knowledge, skills and understanding to make an informed choice about their actions	A programme of education, knowledge and skills to enable clients to choose because they understand the implications. For example, a client may change their diet because they recognise the benefits, not because they are persuaded to change. They are also helped to develop skills such as shopping and cooking
Client-centred or empowerment approach	Clients take control of their own health and establish their goals individually or as a community	Counselling to establish a client's priorities for health or a community's priorities for health
Societal change approach	Physical, social, political or environmental change that promotes a healthy lifestyle	Political and social action such as lobbying for changes in food labelling or action to tackle inequalities

Adapted from Ewles and Simnett (2003)

Naidoo and Wills (2000) have criticised the framework in Table 6.1 for its descriptive approach. Katz *et al.* (2002) add that it is not helpful in identifying why you might select a specific approach or any combination of approaches. Davies and Macdowall (2006) suggest that there are only three approaches to health promotion:

- **Medical and behaviour change** – this focuses on prevention of disease and compliance with diagnosis and treatment.
- **Educational change** – this emphasises that all humans are rational and will change their behaviour to take account of new information they are given.
- **Social change** – this suggests that health is determined by the social, political and cultural environment.

They suggest that these approaches overlap extensively in practice and that their separation into distinct approaches is only useful to highlight their differences. If the approaches are separated, it can lead to oversimplification (see the case study on page 98).

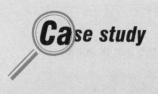

Case study

Sarah's drinking

Sarah is a single parent with three children aged 10–16. She lives in her own house and works full time. Her life is busy and stressful. One way she copes with her stress is to have a glass of wine when she comes home from work. Over time this has increased from one glass to a bottle of wine most nights.

● What do you think would be the most effective approach to help Sarah?

● Would more than one approach be useful?

A medical approach might identify that Sarah is drinking more than the recommended units per day, currently 2–3 units; a glass of wine is 1.5 units (Department of Health 2007). If you combined this with the behaviour change approach, you might be able to empower her to make the decision to change and adhere to the recommended number of units. An educational approach could explore Sarah's knowledge about her alcohol consumption and help her to develop her coping skills.

Taking a client-centred or empowerment approach would help to establish whether Sarah views her behaviour as a problem and could then help her identify ways of coping. A social change approach would recognise the wider issues for Sarah – whether she is getting any support at all from society or is being expected to balance her roles with minimal support.

In reality, one approach cannot address all the issues raised in a situation. The choice of approach or approaches should be dictated by a thorough needs assessment and a clear understanding of the situation. The choice of approach will be influenced by the aims of the health promotion intervention. It is possible to change the approach to suit the situation (Naidoo and Wills 2000).

Over to you

Make some notes on how the approaches in Table 6.1 may be applied to someone in your care.

Health promotion models

Health promotion is complex, so it often helps to use models when you choose your approach and justify your decisions. Do not view the models in isolation and always consider the evidence base for each model. Models are a way of developing practice. They are simplified views of reality that can help in planning, implementing and evaluating programmes (Naidoo and Wills 2000). They are a way of linking ideas and showing the relationship between theory and practice (Ewles and Simnett 2003; Naidoo and Wills 2000).

Models have been criticised: for example, Anderson *et al.* (1999) highlight issues from research into the stages of change model proposed by Prochaska and DiClemente (1982). Although evidence suggests that clinicians can use the Prochaska and DiClemente model reliably and validly, the model does not suggest any strategies that help them move their patients or clients from one stage to the next (Gottwald 2006). There are several models that you could use in your health promotion work. Two popular models are Hochbaum's health belief model (Tones and Green 2004) and Tones's health action model (Tones and Tilford 2001).

Health belief model

The **health belief** model (Figure 6.1) focuses on why people might change their health-related behaviour. Practitioners use it to explain health behaviour through understanding beliefs about health. It suggests that a person bases their health-related behaviour change on four major beliefs (Nutbeam and Harris 2004):

● They are susceptible to the disease or event.

● The disease or event is serious.

● The proposed choices will be successful and prevent the negative event. The benefits of the change outweigh the costs.

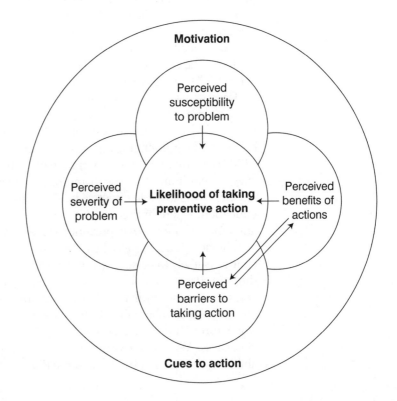

○━┓ Keywords
....

Health beliefs

Health beliefs vary from culture to culture and from person to person within the same culture. They are the elements that a person considers important. Beliefs can be influenced by experiences and can change during a person's life. Education and knowledge can influence beliefs. For example, if you believe it is attractive to be thin, this will influence what you choose to eat. If you believe that smoking helps you relax and improves your mental well-being, you will not be motivated to give up as it could raise your anxiety

Figure 6.1 Health belief model. Adapted from Becker (1974)

If these beliefs are fulfilled, the model predicts that the person will change their behaviour. For example, most parents choose to have their child vaccinated because they think that the advantages of having the vaccination far outweigh any possible side effects from the vaccine (Katz *et al.* 2002). Could a similar example be used to tackle smoking or obesity?

Naidoo and Wills (2000) comment that people's perception of their own risk from a disease is influenced by personal experience, by an ability to control the situation and by their perception of the disease as fatal. They say that people are often overoptimistic about their invulnerability to disease and this makes them unrealistic, which affects the likelihood of their changing behaviour. Tones and Green (2004, p. 81) put it like this: 'Decision making depends on individuals believing that a particular course of action will result in the likelihood of a desired outcome being achieved.'

The health belief model highlights two influences on health behaviour: *cues to action* and *health motivation*. Cues to action are prompts that change health behaviour. Abraham and Sheeran (2005) did a comprehensive evaluation of evidence for the health belief model; they give examples of effective cues to action that have been verified by research. Suppose a family member has developed breast cancer. This may cause others in the family to assess their own risks and change their behaviour and carry out breast self-examination. Another cue to action could be a health promotion campaign that draws an issue to a person's attention such as a reminder about vaccination. Yet another cue could be advice from a health professional, perhaps to give up smoking. A person may receive a cue to action if they notice a change in their health status; for example, breathlessness on exertion may prompt them to quit smoking. A person's motivation towards their own health may influence whether they change their behaviour. This is related to the concept of self-efficacy – whether or not a person believes they can actually change their behaviour.

Rosenstock (1990) suggests some other important mediating variables such as demographics, which includes social class; personality, which is related to self-belief; and structural factors, which indirectly affect behaviour by influencing a person's health beliefs. Nutbeam and Harris (2004) comment on the importance of structural factors when they suggest that limited access to appropriate health-care services and other resources will impede effective health actions. They cite HIV/AIDS education, where limited health-care services and the cost of condoms and other resources may prevent people from changing their behaviour.

The health belief model can help you identify whether an intended change is likely to be successful. For example, does the person believe they are susceptible to a disease or event? How serious do they think it is? Does the person think the change will prevent the disease or event? What are the costs and benefits of the change to the person? If the practitioner works through these questions with a person, it can increase the chances of success. Also consider their motivation, their own assessment of their ability to change and their cue for action.

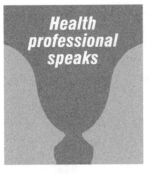

Health professional speaks

Practice nurse

A practice nurse working in health promotion was asked about her use of health promotion models. Here is what she said.

The health belief model helps me assess how people feel about their health and whether they're motivated to change. Before I encourage a person who is obese to adopt a healthy diet or start some exercise, I ask them whether they think they're susceptible to heart disease. I ask if they think they can change then I explore the advantages and disadvantages. I try to find out which aspects they find motivating and which aspects might make them seek support.

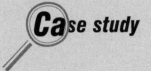

Case study

Adam's blood pressure

Adam is a 45-year-old man. He is married with two children, a boy aged 7 years and a girl aged 9. Until recently, Adam was the chef-owner of a popular noodle bar. His business failed when a hamburger chain opened a restaurant next door to his premises. He cannot raise enough money to open another restaurant but he does not want to work at one of his brother's restaurants. Adam enjoys cooking and he cooks for the family while his wife Sally works full time as a nurse. They live in a high-rise apartment block in East London.

Adam has some health problems. He has become obese since he stopped working. Although he has always smoked, he seems to have increased his consumption since his business failed. He does not like to exercise because he gets breathless after very little exertion. While Adam has been at home he has become less confident in himself and spends a lot of time on his own. Adam attends the local outpatient clinic because he has been feeling dizzy. He has been diagnosed as having high blood pressure. He is anxious about this as his father, who had high blood pressure, had a heart attack and died aged 55. Adam was a young man when his father died and has always felt sad about the lack of time he had with his father.

Answer these six questions, which are linked to the health belief model, to assess whether Adam is likely to change his health-related behaviour.

- Does Adam believe that he is susceptible to a heart attack?
- Does Adam think that a heart attack is serious?
- Does Adam think that the proposed choices will be successful and prevent a heart attack?
- Do the benefits of the change outweigh the costs?
- What are the cues to action?
- Is Adam motivated to change?

The health belief model encourages you to think about Adam's beliefs and consider how to support him to change. He is willing to attend the appointment and appears to recognise that he may be susceptible to an illness, which could be prevented. The model emphasises identifying barriers and benefits and the importance of cues to action, all of which might suggest that Adam will change his behaviour. But this analysis suggests that Adam's lack of self-belief may be preventing any change.

The health belief model can also be used to plan a health promotion programme for a community (see the case study below). The two main ways are to use the model's headings to construct a questionnaire that explores the issues and identifies the community's requirements (Greenwald 2006), or to use the model's headings to inform the planning process and ensure that all the issues are addressed.

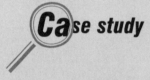

Teenage pregnancies

The national average rate of teenage pregnancy in girls aged 14–16 is 7.8 per 1,000 (Office for National Statistics 2007). You are working in an inner-city area where it is 12 per 1,000. This appears to affect the girls who attend two local secondary schools. Both schools have poor attainment and attendance records for 14–16 year olds. Although this is a national problem, it is particularly significant in this area.

The area has limited facilities for teenagers and it is not seen as cool to visit the local youth club. School is treated as a chore and there is limited engagement. Young people hang around the local park and seem aimless and bored. Many of the young people think that sex is a risk-free activity and few use contraception. The young people place little value on sex and are largely unaware of the consequences of unprotected sex apart from pregnancy. Some of the girls see pregnancy as an acceptable ambition. The area has mixed housing and the unemployment rate is 11 per cent, twice the national average. The area has 30 per cent single-parent households, whereas the national average is 24 per cent.

You have been commissioned to plan a health promotion initiative that will halve under-18 conceptions by 2010.

● Use these headings from the health belief model to help you plan the programme: perceived severity, perceived susceptibility, likelihood of success, benefits of changing, barriers to change, cues to action, motivation.

Applied to the case study above, the health belief model showed that the relevant issue is not just to prevent pregnancies but to help the teenagers value themselves and understand the risks of their behaviour.

Evidence base

Go to the NICE website and read the NICE guidance on how to reduce the conception rate for under-18s. (NICE is the National Institute for Health and Clinical Excellence.)

Support and criticisms

Davies and Macdowall (2006) have highlighted the advantages of the health belief model:

● It is effective in predicting whether a person will adopt preventive strategies or attend for screening.
● It illustrates simply the importance of individual beliefs.
● It highlights the relative costs and benefits of action to improve health.

- Changes in beliefs can lead to changes in behaviour.
- It is a useful tool to help clients assess their own health and manage illness prevention (Roden 2004).

Furthermore it can be used as a planning tool to ensure that beliefs are fully addressed in any health promotion programme (Nutbeam and Harris 2004).

The model has also been criticised:

- One of the major criticisms is that the model focuses on a medical approach to health promotion (Roden 2004). It emphasises a medical view of health as absence of disease rather than a holistic view of health.
- Roden says the model assumes that health-related decisions are rational and conscious. This criticism is backed up by Tones and Green (2004).
- There is little evidence that the model helps to address long-term health issues or issues influenced by social factors such as alcohol misuse and smoking (Davies and Macdowall 2006).
- The model does not acknowledge the wider social determinants of health (Tones and Green 2004). It emphasises individual responsibility and can be seen as blaming individuals for their ill health (Roden 2004).
- The model does not recognise the views of peers and family in influencing individual behaviour (Abraham and Sheeran 2005; Roden 2004).
- The model does not show how its variables are linked to each other or their relative importance in any decision to change (Abraham and Sheeran 2005; Roden 2004).

Despite these criticisms, the health belief model provides a useful framework of issues to consider when planning individual interventions. It is frequently used to help practitioners doing one-to-one health promotion or health promotion in communities (Naidoo and Wills 2000; Nutbeam and Harris 2004; Tones and Green 2004). The health belief model is a relatively simple model that highlights the importance of health beliefs on behaviour. Its credibility is partly based on research which indicates that changes in beliefs can lead to changes in behaviour (Nutbeam and Harris 2004).

Health action model

The health action model (Figure 6.2) was introduced by Tones in the 1970s (Tones and Green 2004). At first sight, it seems more complex than the health belief model, but it is a useful way to analyse whether a health promotion activity is likely to influence a person's intentions. The health action model tries to explain how people make the decision to change their behaviour and what will influence their success.

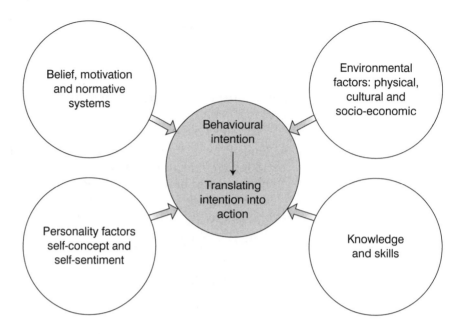

Figure 6.2 Health action model. Adapted from Tones and Tilford (2001)

The first two aspects to consider are behavioural intention and translating intention into action. Behavioural intention is a person's intention to change or to act. The person may want to change their behaviour but whether they actually change depends on a range of factors; for example, a person may want to lose weight and may intend to change their diet but other issues may prevent them. There may be stressors at work or complex personal issues that may impinge on their decision to begin to change their unhealthy behaviour. Translating intention into action is when the person changes their behaviour and sustains this change. This too depends on the person and on factors in their life.

Next come three systems: the belief system, the motivation and the normative system. These systems influence whether a person is likely to translate their intention into action and change their unhealthy behaviours into healthy behaviours. A person may not be able to change their behaviour if their social environment (normative system) means they receive little support from family and friends or if their knowledge and skills (belief system) are inadequate.

- **Belief system** – this is how a person receives information. Taking weight loss as an example, it will be how much the person understands about the importance of weight loss from the factual perspective. It will be influenced by education, information and experience.
- **Motivation system** – this considers a person's value system plus their attitudes and feelings about an issue. Do they value weight loss and is it desirable for them. What do they believe about weight loss? For example, do they believe it will make them happier and healthier or do they believe it will lead to more social relationships?

- **Normative system** – norms are accepted rules of behaviour within a group or society and have cognitive and affective elements. If a person's family are all overweight, it is more difficult for the person to lose weight as being overweight is a norm. If a person's culture values size as an indicator of wealth, it may be more difficult for the person to lose weight.

The first two systems have a reciprocal relationship as information received by a person may create new beliefs. For example, if a person receives information that weight loss increases happiness, they may begin to value weight loss for themselves. But if they strongly believe that weight loss is not a good thing and will make no difference to their lives, this may block any new information.

The health action model also recognises that personality can influence change. In particular, it identifies two areas that are relatively constant, consistent and long-lasting (Tones and Tilford 2001):

- **Self-concept** – this is how the person views themselves, i.e. their self-image, and will include self-efficacy, locus of control and perceived susceptibility.
- **Self-sentiment** – this is linked to self-esteem, i.e. the extent to which people value themselves. This is also associated with temperament and motivation.

The health action model assumes that a person with high self-esteem, an internal locus of control and a positive self-concept will be more likely to perform positive health-related behaviours, whereas a person with low self-esteem and an external locus of control may feel unable to perform positive health-related behaviours for reasons beyond their control (Ewles and Simnett 2003; Katz *et al.* 2002; Tones and Tilford 2001). Self-concept and self-sentiment combine to produce behavioural intention.

A person may intend to change their behaviour but whether they do will depend on factors that sustain change or prevent it. A change can be sustained and become part of the everyday routine, or it can be discontinued and the person relapses back to their unhealthy behaviours. It is important that the nurse or health-care practitioner values a person's decision even if it conflicts with their own values and belief systems. A person may reject suggestions and never initiate an intention. You may find this difficult if your knowledge and skills suggest that behaviour change would be a positive change. To establish a change, the person will need to make a conscious decision. Once the change becomes part of their routine, they will no longer need to make a conscious decision.

An overweight person will need to make conscious decisions to change their diet and choose new foods to eat. Once this has become part of their routine, their eating decisions will become automatic. Health promotion interventions can lead a person to a new behavioural intention, support an existing behavioural intention or have no effect on behavioural intentions.

If an intention is strong, it will require positive factors to help the person reach the action stage. Is the environment supportive to the person or are there physical, cultural and socio-economic barriers. A practitioner needs to identify factors that may support change and those that may not:

- Does the person have the knowledge and skills to initiate and sustain positive health behaviour? For example, do they have the psychomotor skills such as skills to cook healthy food?
- Does the person have the necessary social interaction skills? Can they explain their intentions to their peers and family so they receive support?
- Does the person have self-regulatory skills? Can they monitor their own diet and recognise what they should be eating?
- Is the person able to reinforce the change for themselves and regulate their own drives? Can they devise ways to avoid temptation, identify substitutes and reward themselves so they maintain the new behaviour?

Although the health action model is complex, it does address all aspects of change. It emphasises empowerment and facilitation of positive health behaviours through the development of a person's self-esteem, self-concept and life skills. Nurses and health-care practitioners have a responsibility to work with people to identify their values and beliefs and the things that lead to their unhealthy behaviours. Then they have a responsibility to ensure that people routinely include healthy activities in their lifestyles (Tones and Green 2004).

Over to you

Refer back to the case study on page 101 and use the headings from the health action model to answer these questions that assess whether Adam is likely to translate his intention into action.

- Do Adam's belief, motivation and normative systems prevent him from making the change?
- Does Adam's personality influence his decision and his ability to change?
- Are there strong facilitating factors that will help him translate his intention into action?

Reflective activity

Imagine you are working in the community with a group of young teenagers, as in the case study on page 102.

- Reflect on the health action model and decide whether it would be an appropriate model for planning a programme for these teenagers.
- What would be the advantages and disadvantages of using the health action model when planning a programme for these teenagers?

The health action model is a comprehensive model that gives equal weighting to social situation, personality variables and individual life skills; the health belief model does not go into such depth. The health action model is cited in various texts (Ewles and Simnett 2003; Katz *et al.* 2002; Tones and Green 2004) but there seems to be limited evidence for its effectiveness. Haddock and Burrows (1997) used the health action model in a quasi-experimental design with a small convenience sample of 60 participants. The sample was randomised into a control group or a treatment group. The results showed that 80 per cent of those in the treatment group stopped or reduced their levels of smoking, compared to 50 per cent in the control group. The Haddock and Burrows research also shows that the application of health promotion theory in a programme can affect a person's intention to stop smoking. Despite the apparent lack of research evidence, the health action model remains a useful tool to guide health promotion.

The health belief model and the health action model have shown that the reason why Adam does not change his behaviour is his lack of motivation, confidence and self-esteem, not a lack of knowledge. The practitioners helping Adam need to consider health promotion activities that tackle Adam's lack of motivation, confidence and self-esteem.

Other models

- The stages of change model (Prochaska and DiClemente 1982) explores the process of change and has been used extensively to help people stop smoking (Anderson *et al.* 1999; Aveyard *et al.* 2003; Dijkstra and De Vries 2000; Prochaska *et al.* 2004; Quinlan and McCaul 2000).
- Beattie's model (Earle *et al.* 2007; Naidoo and Wills 2000) helps practitioners to understand the political philosophy that underpins different health promotion activities.
- The theory of reasoned action (Fishbein and Ajzen 1975) is similar to the health belief model and explores beliefs and expectations. It has been used in a variety of programmes, including programmes for exercise promotion (Rivis and Sheeran 2003).
- The health promotion model is a competence- or approach-oriented model that has been used with all age groups and within a variety of cultures (Pender *et al.* 2006).

Choose appropriate models

If you know about a variety of health promotion models, you will be more able to choose an appropriate model as your framework for intervention. The choice of model may also depend on the client's culture, their socio-economic status and their personal values and beliefs.

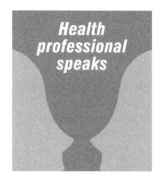

Health visitor

As an experienced health visitor, I often find it helpful to use the stages of change model with clients to establish whether they are ready to quit smoking. Once I have assessed their readiness to quit, it is easier to offer appropriate advice.

Health behaviour

Much health promotion work is based on changes in health behaviour and one of the most popular models is the health belief model, which explains a person's health behaviour by understanding their beliefs about health. Motivational interviewing is a useful technique that you can use as part of the health promotion programme to encourage behaviour change (Miller and Rollnick 2002). This non-confrontational technique differs from the medical approach discussed above and is more in keeping with the client-centred approach. It is useful for those who are somewhat undecided about changing and choose to continue with their unhealthy behaviours (Bonell and Davies 2006; Morrison and Bennett 2006). It has been used with those who have mental health disorders, diabetes and HIV/AIDS, as it is thought to increase insight and compliance with intervention. Motivational interviewing 'allows the person to explore and discover the advantages and disadvantages of their behaviours for themselves' (Rusch and Corrigan 2002, p. 28).

Scaling is a key technique used to explore a person's motivation. Scales are used to find out the importance they attach to a change and their confidence about achieving that change:

- On a scale of 1 to 10 how important is it to give up smoking?
- On a scale of 1 to 10 how confident are you that you could successfully stop?

The points chosen on the scale indicate the person's readiness to change. This is a starting point to explore change, and the practitioner may be able to tip the balance in favour of change by asking questions aimed at increasing motivation and confidence:

- You gave yourself an importance score of 5, why not 1?
- What would need to happen to move you from a 5 to a 7 or a 9?
- What do you think would help your confidence score to move up from 3 to 6?
- How can I help you?

Evidence base

Read Miller, W. R. and Rollnick, S. (2002) *Motivational Interviewing: Preparing People for Change*, 2nd edn. Guilford Press, New York.
Read Rubak, S., Sandboek, A., Luaritzen, T. and Christensen, B. (2005) Motivational interviewing: a systematic review and meta-analysis. *British Journal of General Practice*, **4**, 305–313.

There are clear links between motivational interviewing and health promotion models, especially models of beliefs and attitudes. The main aim of using motivational interviewing is to explore and resolve the ambivalence mentioned above and to reach a resolution that would empower the person to make the decision to change their unhealthy behaviours to healthy behaviours. It is essential that people are empowered to choose, not coerced into a decision (Bonell and Davies 2006). Coercion raises a number of ethical issues. It is essential to respect the ethical principles of beneficence – to do good – and non-maleficence – to do no harm. Questions asked of people could initially relate to the beneficial aspects of their current behaviour and then to the disadvantages. If the positive aspects are considered first, then it is likely that people will gain in confidence and feel more empowered to change (Morrison and Bennett 2006).

Realistic goals and objectives also need to be determined; it is essential to have a caring relationship that includes trust between practitioners and patients or clients (Prochaska and DiClemente 1982). Make your goals and objectives SMART – specific, measurable, achievable, realistic and with a timescale. If the goals are set by practitioner and client together, it may lead to greater achievement and easier evaluation (Tones and Tilford 2001). Make *each* goal SMART. There is no need to have a goal for each letter of the acronym. Setting SMART goals makes it easier to evaluate health promotion programmes easier (Chapter 8).

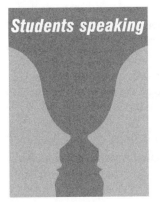

Students speaking

Public health nursing student

When I was working with a woman with diabetes I used some of the principles of motivational interviewing. It was very rewarding to see how she was able to reflect by the end of our sessions and make the decision to begin to change her diet.

Key points **Top tips**

- Show empathy – acceptance facilitates change
- Develop discrepancy – build from within beliefs that change is for the better
- Avoid arguing and generating resistance
- Roll with resistance – reframe negativity, work together to solve problems
- Build confidence – believe in a person's ability to change
- Build on a person's resources, experience and intuition

Health promotion programmes and activities

Health promotion programmes are not new and have been around for 40 years. They address issues of smoking, lack of exercise and raised blood pressure, to name but a few. Changes in these unhealthy behaviours appear to reduce the incidence of heart disease (Morrison and Bennett 2006).

One of the most difficult aspects is to decide which activities to use to empower people to change. The case studies have shown that a key factor is lack of self-esteem, self-efficacy and confidence. Motivational interviewing can facilitate the decision-making process. If self-esteem, self-efficacy and confidence are increased, then stress levels may be reduced. The more people believe themselves to be dealing with the internal and external pressures causing their unhealthy behaviours, the more likely they are to succeed with change. Choose realistic and achievable activities, otherwise the person's self-esteem, self-efficacy and confidence may get even lower.

Choose activities that suit the aim of the programme. If the aim of the programme is to raise awareness, then displays, campaigns and mass media are appropriate. Suppose the aim is to promote healthy eating, then a mass media campaign such as 'five a day' would probably be the most effective. It could also improve knowledge. If the aim of the programme is to change behaviour, then skills training is appropriate, such as training people to select healthy foods, plan a menu and cook a meal. Group work such as social skills training could be included to empower people and develop their assertiveness so they can make the decision to change their diet.

Health promotion can be at the forefront of social change. One example is traffic-light food labelling to distinguish healthy and unhealthy foods. Another example is government policy to improve diet. Wanless (2004) suggested that taxation on unhealthy food might be a way to encourage a healthy diet. He suggested that consumers might make healthier choices if foods high in salt and fat were more expensive, but he acknowledged that dietary choice is complex. He noted that the relationship between a poor diet and health problems such as obesity is not always obvious and he realised that consumers may find ways to avoid the taxes, so higher prices may not promote healthy behaviour. A third example is the healthy school lunch campaign.

Evidence base

Find out about activities to promote a healthy diet at the 5 a day NHS website and the website of Food in Schools.

Evidence-based practice and health promotion

Evidence-based practice focuses on developing practice strategies that are supported by research (Naidoo and Wills 2005). Achieving evidence-based practice requires practitioners to develop their skills in searching for evidence, critical appraisal and applying the evidence in relation to health promotion (Chapter 5). The emphasis on evidence-based health promotion can be related to the worldwide debate on the value of evidence-based practice; be aware of this and base your work on sound evidence (McQueen 2001).

The different health promotion models are supported by different amounts of evidence. One of the difficulties with applying evidence-based practice to health promotion is the dearth of evidence to support the effectiveness of health promotion interventions (Davies and Macdowall 2006). Davies and Macdowall also suggest that the evidence is of variable quality and tends to focus on individual interventions rather than community initiatives. The evidence rarely relates to the process of health promotion or how an intervention works (Naidoo and Wills 2005). The evidence relating to the social determinants of health worldwide is poorly determined (Davies and Macdowall 2006).

Evidence is generally quantitative, which gives some idea of effectiveness but does not explore the wider issues. Evidence may also be from different study designs, such as randomised controlled trials, and different contexts in relation to health promotion and public health. McQueen (2001) argues that there is no agreed hierarchy of evidence for health promotion and that it is essential for health promotion to produce its own hierarchy of evidence due to the complex nature of health promotion and the difficulty in establishing links between cause and effect. McQueen suggests this focus on cause and effect is a reductionist approach to health promotion, and health promotion requires a holistic evidence base as it is a holistic discipline.

But despite these problems there is a need to develop a robust evidence base to support health promotion practice. This is a long-term goal and the process has begun through systematic reviews and public health guidance in a range of subjects. NICE divides public health guidance into two types: public health intervention guidance and public health programme guidance. Public health intervention guidance makes recommendations on types of activities and actions delivered by local health organisations, including recommendations on the types of interventions that should be started or stopped, such as interventions on sexual health and teenage pregnancy (National Institute for Health and Clinical Excellence 2006). Public health programme guidance focuses on how the interventions should be delivered.

The two types of guidance help to achieve the long-term goal of a robust evidence base. Both use a wide range of evidence (Kelly 2006) which recognises the complex nature of health promotion. Guidance will be aimed at practitioners in the NHS as well as in partner agencies and will help address the issues raised above about the nature of evidence and the applicability of evidence-based practice to health promotion.

Conclusion

This chapter has discussed a range of complex issues on interventions to improve health. It defined health promotion and set it in the context of current policy. It explored different levels and approaches to help you identify the most appropriate approach. It described the health belief model and the health action model, applied them to practice and considered the supporting evidence and some of the criticisms. It takes time to change unhealthy behaviour. The chapter suggested some activities that could empower and support people to make the decision to change their unhealthy behaviour and consider healthier lifestyles. It explained the importance of evidence-based health promotion and suggested some strategies to help you overcome the difficulties and challenges. These strategies may be useful ways to promote the health of the people, groups and communities you work with.

Rapid recap

Check your progress so far by working through each of the following questions.
1. Explain the difference between health promotion and health education.
2. What are health beliefs?
3. Define the three levels of health promotion.
4. List and define the different approaches to health promotion.
5. Identify models for health promotion practice.
6. What activities are most useful to help people change their behaviour?

If you have difficulty with more than one of the questions, read through the section again to refresh your understanding before moving on.

References

Abraham, C. and Sheeran, P. (2005) The health belief model. In: *Predicting Health Behaviour*, 2nd edn (eds Conner, M. and Norman, P.). Open University Press, Maidenhead, Berks. pp. 28–81.

Anderson, S., Keller, C. and McGowan, N. (1999) Smoking cessation: the state of the science. The utility of the transtheoretical model in guiding interventions in smoking cessation. *Online Journal of Knowledge Synthesis for Nursing*, **6**, no. 9.

Aveyard, P., Markham, W., Almond, J., Lancashire, E. and Cheng, K. (2003) The risk of smoking in relation to engagement with a school-based smoking intervention. *Social Science and Medicine*, **56**, 869–882.

Becker, M. H. (ed.) (1974) *The Health Belief Model and Personal Health Behavior*. Slack, Thorofare, New Jersey.

Bonell, C. and Davies, M. (2006) *Health Promotion Practice*. Open University Press, Maidenhead, Berks.

Davies, M. and Macdowall, W. (eds) (2006) *Health Promotion Theory*. Open University Press, Maidenhead, Berks.

Department of Health (1999) *Saving Lives: Our Healthier Nation*. HMSO, London.

Department of Health (2000) *The NHS Plan*. HMSO, London.

Department of Health (2004) *Choosing Health*. HMSO, London.

Department of Health (2007) *Alcohol and Health*. www.dh.gov.uk/en/Policyand guidance/Healthandsocialcaretopics/Alcoholmisuse/Alcoholmisusegeneralinformation/ DH_4062199, accessed 10 June 2007.

Dijkstra, A. and De Vries, H. (2000) Subtypes of precontemplating smokers defined by different long-term plans to change their smoking. *Health Education Research*, **15**(4), 423–434.

Earle, S., Lloyd, C., Sidell, M. and Spurr, S. (2007) *Theory and Research in Promoting Public Health*. Sage, London.

Ewles, L. and Simnett, I. (2003) *Promoting Health*, 5th edn. Baillière Tindall, London.

Fishbein, M. and Ajzen, I. (1975) *Belief, Attitude, Intention and Behaviour: An Introduction to Theory and Research*. Addison-Wesley, Reading MA.

Godfrey, C. (2003) Is prevention better than cure? In: Sidell, M., Jones, L., Katz, J., Perberdy, A. and Douglas, A. (eds) (2003) *Debates and Dilemmas in Promoting Health: A Reader*, 2nd edn. Palgrave Macmillan, Basingstoke, Hants, pp. 175–184.

Gottwald, M. (2006) Health promotion models. In: *Rehabilitation: The Use of Theories and Models of Practice* (ed. Davis, S.). Churchill Livingstone, London.

Greenwald, B. (2006) Promoting community awareness of the need for colorectal cancer screening: a pilot study. *Cancer Nursing*, **29**(2), 134–141.

Haddock, J. and Burrows, C. (1997) The role of the nurse in health promotion: an evaluation of a smoking cessation programme in surgical pre-admission clinics. *Journal of Advanced Nursing*, **26**, 1098–1110.

Katz, J., Peberdy, A. and Douglas, J. (2002) *Promoting Health: Knowledge and Practice*. Macmillan, London.

Kelly, M. (2006) Evidence-based health promotion. In: *Health Promotion Theory* (eds Davies, M. and Macdowall, W.). Open University Press, Maidenhead, Berks, pp. 188–194.

McQueen, D. (2001) Strengthening the evidence base for health promotion. *Health Promotion International*, **16**(3), 261–268.

Milio, N. (1986) *Promoting Health through Public Policy*. Canadian Public Health Association, Ottawa.

Miller, W. B. and Rollnick, S. (2002) *Motivational Interviewing. Preparing People for Change*, 2nd edn. Guilford Press, New York.

Morrison, V. and Bennett, P. (2006) *An Introduction to Health Psychology*. Prentice Hall, London.

Naidoo, J. and Wills, J. (2000) *Health Promotion: Foundations for Practice*. Baillière Tindall, London.

Naidoo, J and Wills, J. (2005) *Public Health and Health Promotion: Developing Practice*, 2nd edn. Ballière Tindall, Edinburgh.

National Institute for Health and Clinical Excellence (2006) *About public health guidance*. http://guidance.nice.org.uk/page.aspx?o=295876, accessed 10 June 2007.

Nutbeam, D. and Harris, E. (2004) *Theory in A Nutshell: A Practical Guide to Health Promotion Theories*, 2nd edn. McGraw-Hill, Maidenhead, Berks.

Office for National Statistics (2007) *Conceptions: age of woman at conception*. www.statistics.gov.uk/STATBASE/ssdataset.asp?vlnk=9521, accessed 10 June 2007.

Patient UK (2007) *Health promotion lifestyle*. Patient UK resources on health promotion issues. www.patient.co.uk, accessed 23 February 2007.

Pender, J., Murdaugh, C. and Parsons, M. A. (2006) *Health Promotion in Nursing Practice*. Prentice Hall, Upper Saddle River NJ.

Prochaska, J. and DiClemente, C. (1982) Transtheoretical therapy: towards a more integrative model of change. *Psychotherapy*, **19**, 276–288.

Prochaska, J., Velicer, W., Prochaska, J. and Johnson, J. (2004) Size, consistency, and stability of stage effects for smoking cessation. *Addictive Behaviours*, **29**, 207–213.

Quinlan, K. and McCaul, K. (2000) Matched and mismatched interventions with young adult smokers: testing a stage theory. *Health Psychology*, **19**(2), 165–171.

Rivis, A. and Sheeran, P. (2003) Social influences and the theory of planned behaviour: evidence for a direct relationship between prototypes and young people's exercise behaviour. *Psychology and Health*, **18**, 567–583.

Roden, J. (2004) Validating the revised health belief model for young families. Implications for nurses' health promotion practice. *Nursing and Health Sciences,* **6**(4), 247–250.

Rosenstock, I. (1990) The health belief model: explaining health behaviour through expectancy. In: *Health Behaviour and Health Education: Theory, Research and Practice* (eds Glanz, K., Lewis, F. and Rimer, B.). Jossey Bass, San Francisco, pp. 39–62.

Rubak, S., Sandboek, A., Luaritzen, T. and Christensen, B. (2005) Motivational interviewing: a systematic review and meta-analysis. *British Journal of General Practice*, **4**, 305–313.

Rusch, N. and Corrigan, P. (2002) Motivational interviewing to improve insight and treatment adherence in schizophrenia. *Psychiatric Rehabilitation Journal*, **26**, 23–32.

Sidell, M., Jones, L., Katz, J., Perberdy, A. and Douglas, A. (eds) (2003) *Debates and Dilemmas in Promoting Health: A Reader*, 2nd edn. Palgrave Macmillan, Basingstoke, Hants.

Thibeault, R. and Hebert, M. (1997) A congruent model for health promotion in occupational therapy. *Occupational Therapy International*, **4**(4), 271–293.

Tones, K. and Green, J. (2004) *Health Promotion, Planning and Strategies*. Sage, London.

Tones, K. and Tilford, S. (2001) *Health Promotion: Effectiveness, Efficiency and Equity*. Nelson Thornes, Cheltenham, Glos.

Wanless, D. (2004) *Securing Good Health for the Whole Population*. HMSO, London.

World Health Organization (1986) *Ottawa Charter for Health Promotion*. WHO, Geneva.

7

Working in partnership for public health

Patricia Bond

Learning outcomes

By the end of this chapter you should be able to:

★ Explain what is meant by partnership working in public health

★ Describe different types of partnership approach

★ List the main government policies and initiatives on integrated working in public health

★ Discuss the benefits of partnership working and some of the problems which need to be addressed

★ Identify the essential elements that contribute to a successful partnership

★ Describe and evaluate the strategies that could be used to work in partnership with a community.

Introduction

Working in partnership is about working together to provide fully integrated, easily accessible services based on client or community need and is seen as central to public health policy and practice. It is widely accepted as an important strategic vision and an operational model of practice. Moreover, as rising health-care costs fuel the demand for integrated working in the NHS, the need for coordinated activity and cooperative relationships between agencies and sectors becomes increasingly obvious. Health-care agencies have traditionally worked in isolation, independent from other public service sectors. Inter-agency practice was the exception rather than the rule, but over recent years, **partnerships** have become the dominant model for tackling difficult public health problems (Box 7.1).

The **policy goal** is for statutory, voluntary and private agencies to work in collaboration, either informally or within formalised partnerships, to provide packages of care. This reflects the changing nature of the welfare state and the shift towards services provided by the voluntary and independent sectors.

Partnerships are seen as a means to increase the effectiveness of service delivery, influence other agencies and remedy the inability of single agencies to adequately address the complex health issues of the twenty-first century (Box 7.2). They are also seen as an attempt to overcome the inflexibility of boundaries between service providers, thus making government aspirations for seamless service delivery a more realistic and attainable goal. In fact, the ideal of different agencies working together to resolve complex public health and social care issues has given renewed impetus to the notion of holistic practice.

Box 7.1

Key factors behind the shift to partnership working

- International and national public health policy and changes in legislation from central government
- Appreciation of the wider determinants of health and growing support for population-based core public health functions
- The recognition of complex health needs that cannot be met entirely by a single agency
- Economic necessity, where a single agency cannot afford to fund a project on its own
- Common commitment to a project so that no single agency bears sole responsibility
- The need to enlist community support and enhance user input

Box 7.2

Potential outcomes of good partnership

- Solutions to problems that single agencies cannot resolve
- Promotion of citizen involvement
- Better coordination of services across organisational boundaries
- Avoidance of duplication
- Making best use of available resources

What is partnership working in public health?

Keywords

Partnership
A legal entity governed by law in which the partners accept joint and several liability for their actions and where risk and reward are shared

Policy goals
Goals that reflect the aspirations of a government. They often begin as a political speech or White Paper, but do not receive funding or formal status until they are enshrined in legislation

There is a considerable literature on partnership from a range of academic disciplines, including psychology, sociology, law and the political sciences. This range of interest indicates that contemporary understanding of the term 'partnership' will have different starting points depending on the context. From a public health perspective, Mackereth (2006) describes partnerships as formal or informal relationships among individuals or groups who come together for a common purpose. Harrison *et al.* (2003) adopt a similar position and describe a partnership as people working together towards a shared purpose across services and systems. Sullivan and Skelcher (2002) present partnership as the sharing of responsibility to overcome the inflexibility of organisational boundaries and limited resources. In common, these definitions highlight the need for cooperation between parties in public health to resolve common problems that are unlikely to be solved by the parties working separately. This is a well-rehearsed theme in policy-making circles and is grounded in the view that partnerships develop the capability of organisations and individuals to work across occupational and service divides.

Ultimately, the purpose of partnerships is to harness the synergy of joint working. The Audit Commission (2005) adds weight to this standpoint by broadly characterising partnerships as a formal agreement between two or more independent bodies to work collectively to achieve an objective. This definition draws attention to the additional notion of shared liability. Although not all partnerships in health and social care are legal entities, sharing liability is an important characteristic of partnership working in the commercial sector and increasingly in health and social care, where a partnership agreement may be a condition of funding or a legal duty.

Harrison *et al.* (2003) emphasise that partners will have different motives and power bases. They argue that the ability of the partners to negotiate their position is vital to the success of any partnership, as the mutuality of the union can only be maintained if all parties are able to achieve their own aims as well as the partnership's joint aims. On this point, Eldridge and Martin (2006) suggest that partnership is a pragmatic compromise for participants with different aspirations and power resources. In this regard, White and Grove (2000) propose that effective partnership requires mutual benefits, shared responsibility and shared risks. Moreland *et al.* (2006) add that there must be a strategic fit and the partners must have comparable goals.

In summary, Moreland *et al.* (2006) identify three fundamental types of organisational arrangement that might be described as partnership working (Figure 7.1): joint ventures, where the partners form a new organisation to achieve a defined purpose; strategic partnerships, where partners remain largely separate entities but agree to work collaboratively in a principal area of service development; and comprehensive partnerships, where partners remain legally separate entities but make a commitment to collaborate across interrelated areas on a long-term basis.

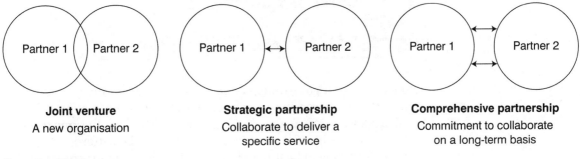

Joint venture
A new organisation

Strategic partnership
Collaborate to deliver a
specific service

Comprehensive partnership
Commitment to collaborate
on a long-term basis

*Figure 7.1 Moreland's
three fundamental types of
organisational arrangement*

Key points **Top tips**

- The term 'partnership' is often used to describe very different collaborative working arrangements. For example, it might be used to describe a professional network of clinicians or to describe a formal arrangement between agencies where budgets for services are 'pooled' under Section 31 of the Health Act 1999.
- Government policy or guidance often advises or prescribes the type of partnership and its responsibilities. Whether the partnership takes executive decisions or functions in an advisory capacity affects its accountability and governance procedures, and this affects its status as a partnership

Over to you

- From your recent work, identify at least three different types of partnership working that you have observed or are involved in.
- List the local factors, national policies and guidance that have been instrumental in the formulation of each partnership.
- Consider how these characteristics influence the status and functioning of the partnership.

How partnership working differs from other working

Despite the popularity of the term, it is not easy to define the essence of partnership. Much confusion and many problems arise from the lack of a uniform definition and the use of interchangeable terms to describe many different working arrangements (Harrison *et al.* 2003). Consequently, it makes sense to explore the differences and similarities that form the range of perspectives on the term 'partnership' in public health.

Reflective activity

Think about how you define partnership working.

Before the Labour government came to power in 1997 and coined the term 'partnership working', other popular phrases were 'teamwork', 'collaboration', 'inter-agency working' and 'networking'. In some texts these terms are still used interchangeably to describe patterns of associated working in health and social care delivery, but increasingly they represent distinct patterns of integration and levels of association.

Each approach is not mutually exclusive, yet there is no straightforward relationship between any of the concepts. Be clear about the differences between the types of associated work, and from this analysis elucidate the key elements of working in partnership. The next section will consider this debate and try to indicate the true meaning of partnership.

Teamworking

Considerable interest has been shown in the concept of teamwork and often the terms 'teamworking' and 'partnership' are used to refer to the same types of interaction. However, teamwork is intrinsically different to partnership and has its own interactional processes, levels of interdependence and coordination of performance. Team members, even across agencies or organisations, tend to conceptualise their work as a shared endeavour. In teamwork there is organised division of labour. Members of a team have a clear collective purpose, such as to win the hockey match or increase productivity. Although individual team members may have specific tasks or roles to complete, there is a sense of equality characterised by reciprocity, mutual hegemony and interdependence. Behavioural and managerial team tasks yield group cohesion, security and attachment. Much of the rationale for teamwork in the health service derives from these benefits.

In this analysis, teams differ fundamentally from partnerships in that members of a partnership may collectively agree goals but they do not override individual goals or ways of working. In addition, team players are judged to be successful when they have achieved their team's goals. A team is best understood in terms of the task it seeks to deliver. Success in partnerships may be measured singularly using individual performance and individual sector or agency targets.

Networking is similar to partnership working but tends to be a more informal way of connecting with people. According to Mackereth (2006), networks are about forming relationships with people to share ideas, link support, and draw on the views and experiences of others. Networks are an important collective identity and help to build a sense of mutuality, common cause and joint action. Hence networks are common in communities and underpin the operation of many self-help groups. Also the term 'networks' gives a better picture of the day-to-day working arrangements of many health and social care practitioners who often don't function in close-knit teams, but work in parallel with each other or cross-refer to other agencies (Ovretveit *et al.* 1997).

Collaboration is also intrinsically different to partnership working but is often used interchangeably with it, most probably because partnership depends on collaboration for its effectiveness (Carnwell and Carson 2005). In common with partnership, collaboration is a process which allows people to work together at different levels (Armitage 1983) and does not exclude participation by the service user. When individuals collaborate, their relationship is based on a desire to pool knowledge and expertise (Soothill *et al.* 1995). In contrast, the purpose of partnership working is not necessarily to pool resources but to better coordinate them to ensure a flexible approach. Parrott (2006) asserts that the term 'partnership' has a stronger connotation than earlier terms such as 'collaboration' and a partnership requires its participants to have much closer and more permanent relationships.

It is possible to distinguish between different approaches to joint working on the basis of their theoretical underpinnings, but it is not always easy to detect differences in practice. So remember that partnership may be based on a mix of ideals. There is no universally accepted definition of partnership, but there are some commonly accepted characteristics (Box 7.3) that may help to identify true partnership. Note that the existence of these characteristics in any partnership is the ideal, rather than the rule. Harrison *et al.* (2003) remind us that many partnerships fall short of the ideal, particularly where the decision to establish a partnership was imposed and did not evolve from a local need.

Box 7.3

Essential elements of partnership working

- Common aims and the acknowledgement of the existence of a shared problem
- An agreed plan of action or strategy to address the problem concerned
- Mutual respect
- Equality
- A cooperative relationship, where individuals gain from each other in an interdependent arrangement
- Collaboration and communication
- Diversity of approach
- Risk taking and shared responsibility

Better services through joint working

The concept of different agencies working together for the common good is not new. What is new is the increased emphasis that government has placed on joint working for public health. When the Labour government came to power in 1997, partnerships were identified as an important way of working to address current health and social care problems. The idea was to breakdown organisational barriers and forge stronger links with local authorities and other service providers who had a role in promoting public health (Department of Health 1997). In addition, there was a goal to promote greater public involvement in health-care delivery so that services were designed around the needs of patients (Department of Health 2000, 2001). A key aspiration was to facilitate the democratic involvement of people in the issues that affect their lives, based on citizenship, shared power, informed choice and autonomy of decision making.

Also, the government's broad agenda to promote social inclusion and community development demanded that agencies and services work together to facilitate long-term planning. One of the six key principles in *The New NHS: Modern, Dependable* (Department of Health 1997) was to involve the NHS in partnership with other agencies to provide health and social care. Health action zones (HAZ) and the New Deal for Communities (NDC) were leading examples of neighbourhood partnerships to tackle health inequalities and modernise services through local innovation and partnership. In HAZ and NDC there is a fundamental commitment to a 'bottom-up' approach, and community partnership was soundly endorsed (Department for the Environment, Transport and the Regions 2001).

Health professional speaks

Community worker

Working in partnership with a community is about engaging people in a vision; it is a mission and the creation of a less bureaucratic way of working. Working in partnership can inspire people locally and empower them to create change. It can galvanise people into wanting to be a part of it. The fact we all share the key vision is critical to making it happen.

The impetus for partnership working was given a further boost by the Health Service Act 1999, which made partnership working a statutory duty for all NHS organisations. Moreover, the NHS Improvement Plan (Department of Health 2004a) outlined priorities up to 2008 and emphasised a commitment to a 10-year process of reform. This improvement plan was significant in that it linked funding to service modernisation, prioritised health service design around the patient, and further emphasised the need for multi-agency working to tackle health inequalities.

To facilitate local partnerships, Department of Health policy also focused on the nature of joint working between health authorities and local authorities. Local strategic partnerships were established specifically to enable local services to work together. Local area agreements (LAAs) made between local and central government also provided a clear framework to help local partners join up and enhance community leadership. More recently the government White Paper *Strong and Prosperous Communities* (Department for Communities and Local Government 2006) outlined plans to improve partnership working and to provide a major expansion of opportunities for local people to influence local decision making.

> ### Over to you
>
> There are three main elements of partnership working in a local area: the local strategic partnership (LSP), the sustainable community strategy (SCS) and the local development framework (LDF):
>
> - Contact your local authority to see if you can locate one or more of these strategy documents.
> - How have these strategies facilitated inter-agency working, community involvement and volunteering in your community?

The government has initiated a raft of cross-government strategies aimed at reducing health inequalities in neighbourhood renewal, employment, education, housing, transport and crime (Office of the Deputy Prime Minister 2005). Although the relationships between the NHS and these wider determinants of health are not necessarily linked in the perception of the general public, factors such as housing, income and employment are considered key determinants of health and well-being (Acheson 1998; Townsend and Davidson 1982; Whitehead 2000).

Ashton and Seymour (1998) recognise that improvements in public health depend more on changes in social and economic policy than on medicine. To improve health, it is essential to involve agencies such as housing, police and education and have them work collaboratively with local communities (Acheson 1998). This has been recognised in the past 15 years of public health strategy, which endorses a multisectoral approach to address the social context of health need and widening inequalities in health. Informed choice, community participation, intersectoral action, and working in partnership to make health everyone's business are key principles of public health strategy in the UK. The emphasis on inter-agency working has therefore been reaffirmed in subsequent public health reviews, including the Wanless Report, which support a multidisciplinary approach to public health provision (Wanless 2002). The White Paper *Choosing Health: Making Healthier Choices Easier* (Department of Health 2004b) recommends building alliances in partnership with local communities. Its main theme underpins the policy view that local communities are the catalyst for change.

> ### Over to you
>
> - Read Chapter 4 of *Choosing Health: Making Healthier Choices Easier* (Department of Health 2004b) and read *Strong and Prosperous Communities* (Department for Communities and Local Government 2006).
> - How far do you agree with the government's view that local community groups can significantly help people make positive health choices?
> - Should communities be given enough power to rebalance the relationship between central government, local government and local people?

Primary care trusts (PCTs) in England have been challenged with converting the rhetoric of intersectoral partnership into public health reality. But many fear that the PCT reconfiguration in 2006 failed to effectively refocus NHS resources because of the impact of the NHS deficit and the slow evolution of commissioning. Nonetheless, under current reforms, there is scope for joint appointments of directors of public health with local authorities, particularly where newly formed PCTs are coterminous with their local authorities. According to Douglas *et al.* (2007), this could place directors of public health in key positions to influence local authority agendas and preserve the intersectoral multidisciplinary initiative.

Making partnership work

Problems in the development of partnerships may not always be apparent at a philosophical level; often partnerships are hampered more explicitly at an operational level. Mundane problems, such as sharing information, communicating with someone with a different perspective from your own, or working across multiple sites, can create barriers to the development of intersectoral partnerships (Table 7.1). To address these potential problems, Harrison *et al.* (2003) suggest that organisational partnerships are treated no differently from any other form of human relationship. They suggest that unless the organisations have previous experience of partnership working, they may need to begin by establishing a basic working relationship.

Table 7.1 Advantages and disadvantages of working in partnership

Advantages	Disadvantages
Access to additional data and information	Overconsumption of resources, especially by smaller agencies
Improved understanding of community needs	Futile attempts to resolve inequalities in boundaries and power
Pooling of resources	Larger agencies tend to dominate and marginalise the objectives of smaller groups
Potential for innovation	Multi-agency strategies are used for face-saving
Opportunities for shared learning	

Evidence base

A really useful model for building effective relationships has been developed by Mead and Ashcroft (2004). Find out more at the Relationships Foundation.

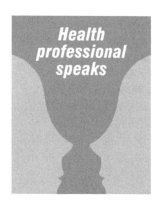

Project manager

Often staff in agencies only find out they are delivering in partnership with another organisation via chance meetings at networks and conferences. Tell all staff about any partnerships that the organisation has developed even if they are not directly involved. This will increase a sense of ownership. Staff need to get to know their partners. How often should they meet? What are the structures needed to share information? How do we deal with dual reporting and arm's-length management? Staff may ask themselves who they have to account to and who will give them support. These issues are not always adequately explained at the outset.

Establish a relationship through good communication

Two prerequisites to relationship building are time for the people in the partnership to get to know each other, and attention to good communication processes and relational skills that put partners at their ease.

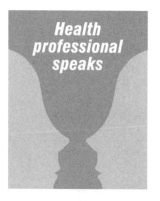

Social worker

A social worker reflects on his partnership working with a child protection agency.

It was initially very personality driven in that we created a very dynamic and keen professional relationship where we worked well together. Dave brings a great deal of clinical experience and we knew that if we could form an effective relationship then it could work. Matt asked lots of questions at the beginning and has a solid background in advocacy, so he brought this to the table and together we have complementary skills and experiences. But we had to do a lot of talking to realise this.

Do not assume that potential partner organisations and their staff understand enough about each other's work, environment and culture to develop a working relationship. The literature suggests that partnerships are more successful when partners relate well to each other and understand each other's roles (Soothill *et al.* 1995). This takes time and is best facilitated by face-to-face contact, informal dialogue and sometimes relationship-building activities. It can also be helpful if people from different organisations come together in small groups to discuss the protocols for working together.

Reflective activity

From your work experiences, think of examples where communication between agencies was good or bad. How did the communication process affect the outcome?

Note that channels and methods of communication will change as the partnership matures. In the early stages, do not make assumptions about other people's information needs. Hornby and Atkins (2000) put the accent on face workers using relational skills such as open listening, empathy and a helping manner to promote understanding. Good communication can also be vital in making contributors feel included and confident. Early in the partnership, spend time on building a communication strategy and schedule regular meetings.

Promote mutual understanding and respect through ground rules

The shift towards partnership working has implications for health professionals, many of whom are not used to this new way of working. Stereotypes and agency subcultures can hinder good working relationships and fuel narrow-minded behaviours and professional rivalries (Carnwell and Buchanan 2005). So there is a need to be informed about each other's roles and to feel comfortable in embracing differences in working practices and styles (Henneman *et al.* 1995). This is not easily achieved, given the predominance of professional cultures supported by uniprofessional training that lacks interdisciplinary opportunities and the techniques to develop teamwork. A particular challenge is to ensure that staff have the necessary skills and knowledge to work flexibly across professional and service boundaries, and the capacity to deal with conflict constructively (Hornby and Atkins 2000). Developing ground rules early on can often enable people to recognise and respect differences, air grievances and manage conflict (Harrison *et al.* 2003).

There are many opinions on what qualities make up an effective partnership but most include respect, trust, honesty and realism (White and Grove 2000). These qualities take time to develop, but by creating conditions where partners feel comfortable to communicate, negotiate and deal constructively with conflict, partnerships will create the optimum conditions for long-term commitment.

Establish robust structures and creative working frameworks

People in partnerships may have to accommodate the organisational needs of their partners and work with organisations for which they have no authority or management responsibility. Partners may also find themselves working together not through choice but as a requirement of government policy or as a condition of funding. When people feel under threat, they come to the relationship feeling cautious and tread tentatively (Harrison *et al.* 2003).

The upshot is that in many partnerships the working territory is uncharted and the opinions varied. Problems can arise where a partnership does not have clear, agreed procedures. Unstructured decision making wastes time, causes conflict and resentments and can lead to partnership breakdown (Ovretveit *et al.* 1997). Developing successful partnerships for that reason depends on dealing with feelings of insecurity and establishing clear boundaries. The challenge is to create the right climate for collaboration.

Sharing of information and resources is difficult in partnerships because of restrictions such as confidential information or processing of personal data. Some information may need to be compartmentalised or ring-fenced, and consents and permissions may need to be re-engineered to facilitate the exchange of information.

Case study

Home-based care for older people

In 2006 a partnership was established between three voluntary care organisations and the local PCT to promote home-based care for older people. It aimed to address service users' social care needs, to reduce the risk of non-elective hospital admission and to improve the use of increasingly limited resources. Each partner was a well-established organisation with its own management and funding. They agreed to work together to provide coordinated social care to older people at risk of hospitalisation from long-term conditions aggravated by social deprivation. An inter-agency steering group was established to support the partnership and coordinate the delivery of a 24-hour telephone helpline plus good-neighbour home visits to at-risk older people.

● What could be the benefits of such a partnership?

● What could be the pitfalls of such a partnership?

● What differences in terminology might arise in a partnership of this type?

● What are the benefits and risks of agencies sharing client information?

To move forward, any partnership has to do a lot of talking about risk scenarios and risk management; it has to agree mutually satisfactory information-governance policies and re-engineer consent processes to facilitate exchange of information in accordance with the Data Protection Act and the Caldicott principles.

> **Over to you**
>
> List the Caldicott principles, available at the Department of Health's website and identify how they apply to your area of work.

Celebrate diversity and guard against inequality

It is easy for large agencies to dominate and stifle the contribution of others. Harrison *et al.* (2003) note that the bureaucratic culture of government-led organisations can be a disincentive to involvement from other sectors. Some small voluntary groups feel that the time, resources and skills needed to function in formal partnerships are too demanding, but nonetheless feel forced into participation by government funding. Equality in partnership can also be difficult to achieve where there are fixed terms and conditions of service delivery plus variations in codes of practice, qualifications and salaries. Moreover, there is a significant danger that small organisations and individuals may feel their contribution is not valued as highly as the contributions of more dominant partners. Harrison *et al.* (2003) claim that smaller voluntary sector organisations may prefer more informal, less structured networks to complex partnerships. To overcome this, partners must seek to emphasise the benefits of diversity, incorporate differences and introduce equal opportunity policies so that groups are not excluded inadvertently.

Promote collective ownership to sustain motivation and commitment

Partnerships that are founded by entrepreneurial individuals may be effective, but if they lack managerial support, they quickly flounder once key personnel leave or move on. To promote collective ownership, partners need to be given authority to become full participants, they need to be clear about the benefits of partnership, and they need to know how long it will take to realise these benefits, so they do not become disillusioned. Partners need to understand the risks and challenges ahead.

Key factors that contribute to successful partnerships

- Partnerships must have an identified important purpose.
- Partnerships need to agree common aims and objectives.
- Partners may need to be innovative and willing to share risks.
- There must be respect, trust and tolerance within the relationship.
- There must be transparency of decision making.
- There must be shared ownership at all levels.
- People representing an agency within a partnership need to know that they have the authority to act on behalf of that agency.
- All partners need to have equal status within the partnership and need to have their contribution acknowledged, whatever their size.
- It may be beneficial to have written agreements for any shared resources.
- Partnerships will need to agree leadership, boundaries, methods of working, lines of accountability and channels of communication.
- Early successes are essential to inspire and motivate long-term commitment.
- Plan for termination of the partnership.

Working in partnership with communities

Working in partnership with communities is fundamental to improving the health of populations and embraces the core principles that are elementary to any community engagement or development activity, principles such as respect for individuals, truth, democracy, fairness and equality.

The steps for working with communities are clearly established (Box 7.4) and share some of the key principles of partnership working. These steps are presented as a sequence but two steps may occur simultaneously or overlap, and some steps may need to be repeated during the life of the partnership.

Box 7.4

Steps for working with communities

1. Identify partners and establish connections with community resources
2. Build relationships
3. Achieve a consensus
4. Encourage community participation
5. Sustain commitment from partners
6. Formulate a partnership agreement and measure success

Step 1 Identify partners and establish connections with community resources

Getting to know and understand your community is an essential first step in creating a community partnership. Chapter 4 described some ways to do this.

First, it is essential to realise that a community is a locality shaped and bounded by its physical geography, amenities, demography, public services, employment, transport, and environment. To work in partnership with a community, you must be cognisant of the features that give it identity. Familiarise yourself with the area and ask key questions about its history, structure and appearance. Local government may define a neighbourhood by the way it organises and delivers its services, and through its civic infrastructure. The area chosen for service delivery may not be coterminous with a neighbourhood where people engage informally. Ascertain whether the area chosen for service delivery has any resonance with the local population as this can inhibit stakeholder engagement and multi-agency working.

Second, the essence of a community is reflected in its social relationships, cultural make-up and level of social contact. When making contact with communities, Twelvetrees (2002) recommends that practitioners should network with social groups by locating faith groups, play groups, youth groups and sports associations and by putting themselves in positions where they will come across people informally.

Step 2 Build relationships

Having gained an understanding of the community, practitioners may establish a relationship with the organisations and individuals they wish to work with. The essence of partnership working is to generate an honest and open relationship in which it is possible to fully understand the range of perspectives in the partnership, and where people feel valued. Much of the work of building a partnership in the community is relatively invisible. Often the emphasis is not on doing but on listening, observing and talking. Here are the important elements of this constructive conversation:

- Think critically.
- Be self-aware.
- Be sensitive to underlying assumptions.

Moreover, to maintain community partnerships, it is crucial to be sensitive to power differentials, particularly when dealing with vulnerable service users. Vulnerable service users may feel unable to assert their preferences and choices for fear of prejudicing their chances of receiving services. It is also possible that community groups may have experienced past encounters that have left a legacy of distrust. The Community Practitioners' and Health Visitors' Association (CPHVA) warns that suspicion and a lack of trust between partners can lead to ineffective working (Mackereth 2006). Meeting in neutral, easily accessible facilities may help ease any potential tensions.

Step 3 Achieve a consensus

It is unrealistic to assume that all sections of a community share the same values and priorities. Local communities are not homogeneous entities. They consist of groups with interrelated differences, including gender, age, religion, ethnicity, wealth and local interests. In practice, client participation in community partnerships requires the selection of community representatives. Attempts at representation without careful consideration may smack of tokenism or may even become biased if the needs of the whole community are poorly represented. In addition, many attempts at representation lack any formal accountability mechanisms to ensure the opinions voiced are valid expressions of the local community. Therefore important decisions have to be made about which clients participate, on whose behalf they participate, and how they are chosen.

Successful partnerships seek to balance the needs and expectations of critical stakeholders. Not all stakeholders have equal importance in each situation and it is up to the partnership manager to ensure that the views of people in a partnership are balanced at appropriate times. For example, in a school-based obesity programme where health agencies seek to work in partnership with schools, the views of parents, teachers and school governors are critical to the partnership's success, but students are unlikely to participate if they feel embarrassed or degraded by the programme. Problems may arise when powerful stakeholders have conflicting expectations of the partnership. Carefully consider the potential differences in stakeholder views, and focus early discussion on areas of compromise and reconciliation.

Step 4 Encourage community participation

Social groups can be a useful staring point for partnership work. Associations such as schools, churches, sports clubs and other forms of community group function in two ways. Firstly, they act as social networks by enhancing the interaction of members with each other. Second, they serve as mediating structures between individuals and larger public institutions. These associations combine the identities of members and represent them as a collective to the outside world. Most community associations typical of those described above are highly adept at representing the voices of people who may be marginalised. Forming relationships with these groups is fundamental for community capacity building. According to Arnstein (1969), true participation involves delegated power and citizen control. The role of the public health practitioner in facilitating community participation lies in mobilising people to take an active part in the delivery of services.

The public health nurse must guard against oversimplified processes of engagement such as consultation. Consultation is the process of seeking information, advice, opinions and perspectives from individuals, groups and communities. In the consultation process, the consulted usually have a formal role in expressing their views and experiences; they have a right to be heard, but they do not take an active part in the partnership's decision making. The aim of their involvement is to modify existing systems to meet local needs but the major influence still rests with the professionals. In partnership the goal is to shift the balance of power to promote equality in the decision-making process. At a very basic level, partnerships provide the infrastructure needed for consultation, but in the context of a community initiative they can ensure community representatives are actively involved in decision making. A partnership agreement co-opts community representatives into policy decision making and gives them equal status with the professionals. Box 7.5 lists the prerequisites for promoting participation.

Box 7.5

Prerequisites for promoting participation

- Disseminate information about the proposed partnership through local champions, community representatives, outreach nurses, and local outlets such as shops, community centres and youth clubs
- Be aware of basic access needs, including wheelchair access, sign language services and translation facilities, as well as the religious and cultural observations of specific user groups
- Formulate service agreements, communication plans and payment protocols to facilitate individual engagement
- Develop members of the community so they have the confidence and skills to represent the views of the community
- Empower people with advice, language services and advocacy

Reflective activity

Think about the community you work with and list the ways you have used to encourage participation.

Step 5 Sustain commitment from partners

To achieve the goals of community development, all parties need to stay committed to the partnership process. They need to acknowledge that participation has its costs in time, energy and possibly money. All parties need to understand what really motivates people to participate in community partnerships and what facilitates collective action. Findings suggests that people living in deprived communities are less likely to engage in community partnerships because they lack the self-confidence, have competing social agendas, and have a tendency to resolve problems on their own with little recourse to community support. Incentives are essential to sustain partnership working. Make it clear from the outset how the service user will be reimbursed for their participation, and, as the partnership develops, make the benefits comparable with local need.

To maintain their interest and level of engagement, user groups may need help to articulate their needs and to break away from an attitude where they expect professionals to provide services. For many social groups, partnership is experienced simply as a consultation process where there is co-option into the decision-making process. Consequently, people become fatigued by participatory activities such as steering groups, focus groups, questionnaires and citizens' juries and come to realise that they do not alter their core needs. The ultimate purpose of capacity-building activities within a partnership is to rectify this situation by incorporating community representatives more deeply into partnership decision-making processes and to facilitate shared responsibility, where both parties contribute resources and share risks. The payback then comes in a sense of ownership, renewed empowerment and control.

Step 6 Formulate a partnership agreement and measure success

An essential part of forming a partnership is about making working arrangements explicit, detailed, unambiguous and sometimes formal. A written agreement between agencies and users is an essential stepping stone in making a full and honest commitment to the partnership. It is often a prerequisite to gaining resources and applying for funding. Partnership agreements are useful tools for evaluation as they clearly set out objectives, timetabled actions, channels of communication, resources, personnel and outcome indicators. Decisions about when and how to evaluate will depend on the purpose of the partnership, the availability of the outcome data and the views of the commissioners. Outcomes are evaluated at the end of a partnership. There are a range of options and tools for outcome evaluation: questionnaires, work diaries and participant observation. For many professionals, evaluation of partnership working is all about measuring processes and gaining feedback. If this is the case, when the partnership is created, the partners should build in an action research approach to evaluation. An **action research** approach has the advantage of allowing the project to be improved as it develops.

⊶ *Keywords*

Action research
The term 'action research' is thought to be the creation of Kurt Lewin, an early 20th century psychologist and philosopher. He recognised a need for a form of research that would lead to social action. His approach involved a cycle of planning, action and fact finding about a problem in practice. Health programmes are increasingly using action research and the Department of Health has recommended it as a valuable method in health research

Recognise the role of service users as partners

Over the past decade, partnership with patients and clients has clearly evolved so that disadvantaged and traditionally less vocal citizens, such as the homeless, people with a disability and people with mental health problems, have been helped by the consumerist movement to demand a greater say in their own care (Ferrant 1991; Saltmann 1994). Policy changes during the 1990s led to greater patient or client choice and, most important, greater user representation in service commissioning, design and evaluation. Besides these changes, greater access to authoritative health-care information has changed the balance of power in patient–practitioner relationships. Commentators note the movement to more participatory patient–practitioner relationships and the rise of client involvement, co-service delivery and participation in service delivery. New terms have evolved that give better descriptions of people accessing health care in the UK. Terms such as 'user', 'client' and 'consumer' are now commonplace and help practitioners rethink their relationship with the people they serve. The casual observer might conclude that service providers have come a long way in translating the partnership ideal into practice, but what do users think?

Reflections on the process of partnership working by service users paint a disappointing picture. Many users emphasise feelings of powerlessness, mechanistic service delivery arrangements that fail to take account of personal preferences, and impenetrable, bureaucratic organisations that require skill, ingenuity and creativity to access. One reason for these negative feelings is that partnership implies a level of equality between partners that still does not exist. Citing the experiences of informal carers working across the interface of formal and informal care, Chambers and Philips (2005) argue that informal carers do not have access to the power and resources available to formal carers, which puts them at a constant disadvantage.

Chambers and Philips (2005) suggest that professional stereotyping and paternalism exacerbate service users' perceptions of powerlessness. A key failing is not recognising that service users and carers are individuals and citizens with a multiplicity of roles and responsibilities. Few service users are reimbursed for their contribution to service planning and they are seldom offered direct employment. Moreover, professionals rarely see service users as co-workers. On this point, Eldridge and Martin (2006) claim that the name 'service user' highlights the essence of the problem. The implication in the name is that the service user has a need that is satisfied by service providers. Eldridge and Martin (2006) explain that this does not suggest a relationship that is mutually beneficial or equal. This critique has led to the development of the 'expert patient' and 'carers as experts' programmes.

This chapter began by describing partnerships as capable of generating a fertile space where new perspectives could take root. But partnership working remains a challenge for people with stigmatising diseases such as HIV/Aids or mental illness. Reviewing the involvement of hard-to-reach groups, Sullivan and Skelcher (2002) suggest that even where projects have actively targeted minority or marginalised groups, their success has been minimal, and many groups remain on the periphery of the partnership process.

Social attitudes towards some marginalised groups such as illicit drug users, young offenders or prisoners send contradictory messages to health-care professionals about working in partnership. The partnership is often problematic because there is a difficult balance between being an ally, risk management and public protection. Moreover, service providers may vary considerably in their assessments of the risks posed by different groups, which makes inter-agency partnership even more problematic. For example, a drug-using mother could discuss her drug habit with her GP, health visitor, probation officer, social worker or housing officer. Each may have a different view of the risks posed by her habit, based on theoretical, philosophical and professional differences. Buchanan and Corby (2005) support this view and claim that policy and practice on drug misuse and child protection too often remain parochial and uncoordinated. Eldridge and Martin (2006) add that the media and socio-political pressures stimulate an increasingly paternalistic and controlling approach that is incompatible with equity and trust in a partnership and reinforces the idea of powerlessness in the minds of the service users.

An overriding assumption of the partnership movement is that users wish to be partners in their care. But a person's readiness to work in partnership is influenced by past experiences as well as society's expectations. To sustain true partnership, front-line workers need to be sensitive to their clients' and carers' needs and to recognise that stereotypes, gender roles and other prejudices may hinder the collaborative process.

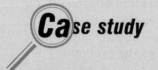
Case study

Elsie and Alan

Elsie is 75 and lives with her husband, Alan, in their one-bedroom bungalow. They have one daughter who lives 16 km away. Elsie suffers from multiple sclerosis (MS) and is wheelchair bound.

Before Elsie deteriorated, she could use her wheelchair to get to the bathroom door, then she could reach the shower by using a frame; her feet still had some mobility. Alan used to wash and comb her hair and helped to choose her clothes each day. When Elsie deteriorated, social services asked care workers to make regular visits to her house. They were very diligent and dressed and washed Elsie twice a day. They even helped her choose her clothes and took laundry away for washing.

Alan was grateful for the help but felt very alone and excluded. He had cared for his wife all his life and longed to be able to care for her again. He felt angry that the care workers had taken away his caring roles and felt they had excluded him because of his gender. Elsie didn't want Alan to raise the issue because she was concerned about how her new carers would react.

- To what extent do you think that stereotypes and gender roles get in the way of the rights of informal carers?

- Do you think Alan was justified in his feelings?

- If you were one of the care workers in this scenario, how would you have worked in partnership with Alan and Elsie?

Conclusion

Public health service planning, delivery and evaluation are increasingly based on partnerships insofar as there is an obligation for collaboration between different public sectors, professionals and user groups. The idea that joint working enhances public service is the cornerstone of contemporary health and social care policy. Collaboration through partnerships between public sector agencies and professional disciplines has been trumpeted as the way forward to bring down the Berlin Wall dividing health and social care. The involvement of communities and service users within these newly constructed working arrangements appears to add legitimacy to this process. But partnership working is not easy and is not a panacea for the economic challenges of multifaceted health need. Redefining practice boundaries in the context of partnerships will have significant implications for those professionals in health and welfare services who are accustomed to working exclusively within the margins of their own organisation.

A particular challenge is to ensure that practitioners and service users have the knowledge, skills, attitudes and values to work flexibly across occupational and service boundaries. This chapter has elucidated the concept of partnership and examined the context and processes of partnership working. For practitioners new to public health, it highlighted some of the essential values, skills and attitudes involved, and explained how they can be translated into the process of partnership working with communities. The challenges and benefits of partnership working were presented to help prepare new practitioners for the reality of collaboration. To remain authentically in partnership, a practitioner needs to be honest and open in their communication, and reflective in their practice.

RRRR*Rapid recap*

Check your progress so far by working through each of the following questions.

1. List three potential outcomes of a good partnership.
2. Name three characteristics that define a high-quality partnership.
3. Identify the key drivers that underpin the shift towards integrated working.
4. What are the key steps in making partnership work?

If you have difficulty with more than one of the questions, read through the section again to refresh your understanding before moving on.

References

Acheson, D. (1998) *Independent Inquiry into Inequality in Health: Report*. HMSO, London.

Armitage, N. H. (1983) Joint working in primary health care. *Nursing Times*, **79**, 75–78.

Arnstein, S. R. (1969) A ladder of citizen participation. *Journal of the American Institute of Planners*, **35**(4), 216–224.

Ashton, J. and Seymour, H. (1988) *The New Public Health*. Open University Press, Milton Keynes, Bucks.

Audit Commission (2005) *Governing Partnerships: Bridging the Accountability Gap*. Audit Commission, London.

Buchanan, J. and Corby, B. (2005) Drug misuse and safeguarding children: a multi agency approach. In: *Effective Practice in Health and Social Care: A Partnership Approach* (eds Carnwell, R. and Buchanan, J.). Open University Press, Maidenhead, Berks.

Carnwell, R. and Buchanan, J. (eds) (2005) *Effective Practice in Health and Social Care: A Partnership Approach*. Open University Press, Maidenhead, Berks.

Carnwell, R. and Carson, A. (2005) Understanding Partnerships and Collaboration. In: *Effective Practice in Health and Social Care: A Partnership Approach* (eds Carnwell, R. and Buchanan, J.). Open University Press, Maidenhead, Berks.

Chambers, P. and Phillips, J. (2005) Working across the interface of formal and informal care of older people. In: *Effective Practice in Health and Social Care: A Partnership Approach* (eds Carnwell, R. and Buchanan, J.). Open University Press, Maidenhead, Berks.

Department for Communities and Local Government (2006) *Strong and Prosperous Communities: The Local Government White Paper*. HMSO, London.

Department for the Environment, Transport and the Regions (2001) *New Deal for Communities. Annual Review, 2000–2001*. DETR, London.

Department of Health (1997) *The New NHS: Modern, Dependable*. HMSO, London.

Department of Health (2000) *The NHS Plan*. HMSO, London.

Department of Health (2001) *Involving Patients and the Public in Health Care*. HMSO, London.

Department of Health (2004a) *The NHS Improvement Plan: Putting People into the Heart of Public Services*. HMSO, London.

Department of Health (2004b) *Choosing Health: Making Healthier Choices Easier*. HMSO, London.

Douglas, J., Earle, S., Handsley, S., Lloyd, E. and Spurr, S. (2007) *A Reader in Promoting Public Health*. Sage, London.

Eldridge, K. and Martin, P. (2006) *Partnerships in Health*. Quay Books, London.

Ferrant, W. (1991) Addressing the contradictions in health promotion and community action in the United Kingdom. *International Journal of Health Sciences*, **21**(3), 423–439.

Harrison, R., Mann, G., Murphy, M. and Thompson, N. (eds) (2003) *Partnership Made Painless: A Joined-Up Guide to Working Together*. Russell House, Lyme Regis, Dorset.

Henneman, E. A., Lee, J. L. and Cohen, J. (1995) Collaboration: a concept analysis. *Journal of Advanced Nursing*, **21**, 103–109.

Hornby, S. and Atkins, J. (2000) *Collaborative Care*. Blackwell, Oxford.

Mackereth, C. J. (2006) *Community Development: New Challenges, New Opportunities*. Amicus, London.

Mead, J. and Ashcroft, J. (2004) Relationships in the NHS: bridging the gap. Discussion document, www.relationshipsfoundation.org, accessed March 2007.

Moreland, N., Jolley, D., Read, K. and Clarke, M. (2006) Partnership and capacity building for African-Caribbean and Asian elders with dementia. In: *Effective Practice in Health and Social Care: A Partnership Approach* (eds Carnwell, R. and Buchanan, J.). Open University Press, Maidenhead, Berks.

Office of the Deputy Prime Minister (2005) *Creating Healthier Communities: A Resource Pack for Local Partnerships.* ODPM, Wetherby, Yorks.

Ovretveit, J., Mathias, P. and Thompson, T. (eds) (1997) *Inter-professional Working for Health and Social Care.* Macmillan, London.

Parrott, L. (2006) The political drivers of working in partnership. In: *Effective Practice in Health and Social Care: A Partnership Approach* (eds Carnwell, R. and Buchanan, J.). Open University Press, Maidenhead, Berks.

Saltmann, R. (1994) Patient choice and patient empowerment in northern European health systems: a conceptual framework. *International Journal of Health Services*, **24**(2), 201–229.

Soothill, K., Mackay, L. and Webb, C. (eds) (1995) *Inter-professional Relations in Health Care.* Arnold, London.

Sullivan, H. and Skelcher, C. (2002) *Working Across Boundaries: Collaboration in Public Services.* Palgrave Macmillan, London.

Townsend, P. and Davidson, N. (1982) *Inequalities in Health: The Black Report.* Penguin, Harmondsworth, Middlesex.

Twelvetrees, A. (2002) *Community Work*, 3rd edn. Palgrave, Basingstoke, Hants.

Wanless, D. (2002) *Securing Our Future Health: Taking a Long-Term View.* HMSO, London.

White, K. and Grove, M. (2000) Towards an understanding of partnership. *NCVCCO Outlook*, no. 7.

Whitehead, M. (2000) *The Health Divide.* Health Education Council, London.

8
Evaluating public health approaches

Sue Rouse and **Yvonne Wilkinson**

Learning outcomes

By the end of this chapter you should be able to:

★ Explore the concept of evaluation in the context of public health

★ Discuss a range of methods that could be used to evaluate public health interventions

★ Select an appropriate method of evaluation for a range of public health approaches.

What is evaluation?

In a time of limited NHS resources, it is essential to have evidence about the effectiveness of all types of intervention. However, evaluations of public health initiatives in nursing and health-care practice appear to be scarce; most evidence focuses on the medical aspects, which can often be more readily evaluated and proved to be effective (Plews *et al.* 2000). Evaluation of public health interventions has been acknowledged as difficult, partly due to the positive concept of health that is used by practitioners and which appears to be at odds with the more usual disease focus of the NHS. Robinson reported the interpersonal element of the role or the relationship-centred approach that is deemed to be difficult to quantify or measure (Craig and Smith 1998). Evaluation is a difficult but necessary task for practitioners; this chapter considers some ways to do it.

Evaluation in its purest form can be defined as a 'judgement of the value of something' (Ewles and Simnett 1999, p.88). This succinct definition could be seen as too simplistic in an increasingly competitive NHS environment, where efficiency and effectiveness are integral requirements. So let us consider some more detailed definitions. From an educationalist perspective, Neary (2000) suggests that evaluation is a systematic collection and analysis of information about how successful a programme has been as part of a student's learning experience. Polit and Hungler (1993) suggest that evaluation research is an investigation into how well a programme, practice or policy is working.

There are many definitions of 'evaluation' but they all contain the idea of assessing whether goals have been achieved and assessing the effects of an intervention. Green and South (2006) state that evaluation is concerned with assessing what has been achieved and identifying how any changes have come about. This suggests that evaluation can be seen as having two elements, often known as outcome evaluation and process evaluation. But there is no single defining set of terminology for these two elements. Several other terms are used for outcome evaluation, such as summative evaluation, impact evaluation and output evaluation. Output evaluation is often associated with the materials and activities that are produced to achieve the outcomes; it aligns itself to process evaluation, which is also called formative evaluation.

Outcome evaluation is concerned with what has been achieved and whether goals or aims have been met. Process or output evaluation is concerned with how things have been achieved, whether the most appropriate resources were used, and whether the method used was the most effective. Outcome evaluation is seen as an evaluation of the end product whereas process evaluation examines the approach used to deliver the end product. Outcome evaluation and process evaluation can be achieved by several approaches using quantitative and qualitative methods.

The purpose of evaluation

The concept of evaluation should already be familiar to nurses and health-care practitioners who have used *The Nursing Process* (General Nursing Council 1977; Yura and Walsh 1967) or similar to underpin their approach to practice. The concept of a systematic approach to practice comprising assessment, planning, intervention and evaluation encourages practitioners to compare the actual behaviours of patients or clients at a particular point in their care with the goals previously set (Aggleton and Chalmers 1986). Following this systematic approach, evaluation fits into the public health cycle (Figure 8.1). In this way, the first purpose of evaluation can be identified as assessing effectiveness through determining the extent to which goals have been met.

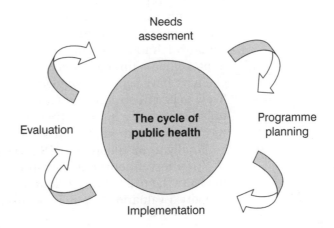

Figure 8.1 Evaluation is one stage in the cycle of public health

Reflective activity

Think about a patient or client care plan you are currently involved with:

- What are the goals or objectives of your planned care?
- Where and how are your goals recorded?
- How will you know whether you are achieving your goals?
- How will you record what you have achieved?
- What will happen to the information you gather?

The use of evaluation to determine effectiveness implies the need to set clear goals at the planning stage of any intervention, including public health interventions. The nature of the goals will be determined by the approach to public health. For example, a behaviour change approach should produce some measurable change in behaviour whereas an educational approach should lead to a change in knowledge and attitude as well as a change in behaviour. These ideas will be explored further later in this chapter.

A second purpose of evaluation develops the theme of assessing effectiveness. Once it has been established that a chosen method of implementing a public health intervention has been successful in meeting some predetermined goals, this forms the beginnings of an evidence base of what works. Although not necessarily conforming to the requirements of formal quantitative research, routine evaluation of service outcomes produces some valuable data relating to the establishment of an evidence base for public health practice. Indeed the role of England's Health Development Agency includes 'maintaining an up-to-date map of the evidence base for public health and health improvement' (Department of Health 2001a). Naidoo and Wills (2000, p.297) define such an evidence base as 'the sum total of research evidence that suggests which health initiatives are likely to succeed if replicated in other populations or geographical areas'.

Thirdly, evaluation of public health interventions and the establishment of an evidence base lead to valuable learning about which interventions are effective, and this informs service improvements through effective dissemination and implementation. Once we have some knowledge about which types of intervention are likely to be effective, we can apply the knowledge to improve our own practice and pass it on to others to help them improve theirs. In this way, service users will benefit from continuous service improvement.

Finally, as for all other NHS services, there is a need for public health interventions to demonstrate cost-effectiveness in order to justify the use of finite resources or to seek further financial support. Evaluation of public health interventions can demonstrate the achievement of outcomes that relate to the delay or prevention of morbidity or mortality; for example, reducing the prevalence of cigarette smoking can reduce the incidence of lung cancer. This in turn may lead to cost reductions in treatment interventions. Favourable comparisons between the cost of the public health intervention and the consequent savings in treatment costs can contribute to evidence of cost-effectiveness.

Furthermore, there is the potential to demonstrate cost-effectiveness not only in relation to financial resources, but also in terms of human pain and suffering resulting from morbidity or early mortality.

Key points | Top tips

Evaluation of public health interventions has four related purposes:

- to determine the effectiveness of individual interventions in relation to defined goals or objectives
- to develop an evidence base about which interventions are more likely to be effective in a given set of circumstances
- to improve services through implementation of interventions with proven effectiveness
- to demonstrate cost-effectiveness to inform prudent use of finite NHS resources

Approaches to evaluation

Evaluation is an essential and integral part of any public health intervention. There are several evaluation approaches. The choice of approach largely depends on the type and purpose of the public health intervention.

Evidence base

Read Elkan, R., Mitch, B. and Robinson, J. (2000) Evidence-based practice and health visiting: the need for theoretical underpinnings for evaluation. *Journal of Advanced Nursing*, **31**(6), 1316–1323.

Randomised control trials

Randomised controlled trials (RCTs) are seen as the classic experimental method and the gold standard in quantitative evaluation (Bowling 2002). In their simplest form, they involve a sample population with similar characteristics that is randomly allocated to the intervention group or the control group. The intervention and control groups are carefully monitored to minimise any variation between them and data is collected and analysed to establish the statistical significance of the intervention's effects. RCTs are usually associated with research activity. Although there are similarities between research and evaluation, there are some distinctions: research focuses on determining an evidence base for practice whereas evaluation is primarily concerned with measuring the effectiveness and efficiency of practice and the achievement of defined goals.

An example of how this methodology could be employed is in evaluating the effectiveness of different types of vaccination preparations, such as comparing the outcomes of combined diphtheria, tetanus and pertussis vaccination (control group) with those of individual vaccinations (intervention group). This approach strongly aligns itself with the medical model of health care (Glasgow *et al.* 1999). However, RCTs can be used in the broader public health arena to determine best practice and evaluate the effectiveness of different interventions. For example, in relation to smoking cessation the control group may take nicotine replacement therapy (NRT) and the intervention group may have NRT and counselling once a week for 3 months. This would determine whether smoking cessation therapy with NRT and counselling is more effective than NRT therapy alone.

There are potential problems with the use of RCTs to evaluate public health initiatives. It could be suggested that RCTs fail to consider the wider determinants of health, the complexities of public health and how health behaviour is determined. Tones and Green (2004, p.327) suggest that 'control within communities is difficult to maintain and is often contaminated'. Therefore other approaches may be more appropriate for evaluating public health practice.

Questionnaires

Questionnaires can also be used within a quantitative approach to evaluation and are seen as experimental in design; they are useful in collecting information from relatively large numbers of people and smaller groups. There needs to be careful consideration given to the design of the questionnaire and the formulation of questions to provide valid conclusions. To avoid ambiguity, keep questionnaires as simple as possible (Bowling 2002; Ewles and Simnett 1999). Public health practice uses pre–post questionnaires for evaluation, such as in a school-based health education programme that aims to increase awareness of binge drinking among schoolchildren.

In a pre–post approach, levels of awareness can be measured using questionnaires before and after the programme to assess its effectiveness. But even if the findings show an increase in awareness, it is inappropriate to attribute the increase entirely to the health education programme. Pupils may have sought further information from their peers, magazines and television in response to the topic being highlighted. Ultimately, it could be argued, the increase may also be due to the intervention sparking that interest, so it should be seen as an integral part of evaluation, not something which detracts from it. These sorts of external influence form part of the complexity of public health. People do not make health choices in a vacuum but in response to external pressures in the context of the wider environment (Naidoo and Wills 2000).

Over to you

Read Chapter 12 in Bowling (2002) on questionnaire design.

- What are the two most important aspects in constructing a questionnaire?
- Why would you choose to use open-ended questions? Give an example of an open-ended question.
- Why would you choose to use closed questions? Give an example of a closed question.

Some advantages of questionnaires are that they are suitable for large and small groups; anonymous questionnaires may mean that respondents are more truthful; and they can provide an instant or more long-term evaluation depending on how they are used. Some disadvantages of questionnaires are that their response rates are often low, so they do not give an accurate evaluation of the public health intervention; and their questions may be interpreted differently from intended. Piloting the questionnaire with a smaller group may help to avoid some of the disadvantages. Questionnaires may also be supported by other evaluation methods such as interviews; this gives the evaluation a quantitative element and a qualitative element.

Statistical analysis of other data types

Statistical analysis is not exclusively for RCTs. It may be used to evaluate other public health data. A vast amount of statistical data is collected on NHS departments and other agencies, such as employment, education, social services and housing. This data can be analysed to evaluate public health initiatives. For example, to improve the immunisation rate of schoolchildren in a rural area, practitioners may set up an immunisation session in a school. The need may have been identified partly by analysing the low immunisation rates provided by the child health department. Following the immunisation session in the school, the immunisation statistics could be evaluated to determine its effectiveness.

o—ᴛ *Keywords*
....

Structured interview
An interview that uses
prepared questions

**Semi-structured
interview**
An interview based
on identified areas for
discussion or exploration

Unstructured interview
An interview on a defined
topic but where there is no
defined structure for the
interview content or flow

Interviews

RCTs and questionnaires are quantitative evaluations and use a
statistical approach, but they can be limiting and may need to be
supplemented with a qualitative evaluation. Qualitative evaluation
focuses on the meanings that people attach to their social world
and attempts to capture the subjectivity of human beings (Bowling
2002). Green and South (2006) suggest that complex public health
interventions do not conform to a simple input–output model of
evaluation, so they need to be evaluated using both qualitative and
quantitative methods. Interviews can be done with one person or
a group of people, such as a focus group or community group; they
can provide in-depth evaluation of the outcome and the process of
the intervention. Interviews can be **structured**, **semi-structured**
or **unstructured** (Bowling 2002).

The advantages of interviews are that they gather in-depth
information; the interviewer and interviewee can give clarification,
which is impossible with a questionnaire; and they can elicit
unexpected but highly relevant information. Some disadvantages of
interviewing are that it is often time-consuming and interviewees
may give responses that are intended to please the interviewer,
especially if a rapport develops during the interview. Interviewers
should pay attention to the interview questions and try to avoid
biasing or leading the interviewee's responses; they should
accurately record and report the interviewee's views so that valid
conclusions can be drawn.

Formal interviews can be conducted at the end of the intervention
to evaluate the outcomes. Formal or informal interviews during the
course of the intervention may be used to evaluate the intervention
process. For example, participants in a stress management group
were interviewed part-way through the programme; the interviews
highlighted dissatisfaction with the programme's content and
format. Interview feedback allows an intervention to be adjusted to
make it more effective.

Informal feedback

Informal feedback is an important element of outcome and process
evaluation, but it is more commonly associated with process
evaluation. Throughout an intervention, encourage written, verbal
and non-verbal feedback from clients, colleagues and stakeholders.
Informal feedback can provide in-depth data. Analyse the data
constructively and use it to improve the intervention (Neary 2000).
To encourage feedback, practitioners need to be accessible and
create an atmosphere of openness and honesty (Ewles and Simnett
1999).

Reflective activity

Think of a situation where you have received feedback from a colleague, patient or client. How did it feel? Was it useful? Did you think the feedback was open and honest? On reflection, would you have delivered it differently? If so, how?

Observation

Another method of evaluation is direct observation of behaviours during and after an intervention. For example, the safe disposal of needles and syringes by drug users could be evaluated by observing a decrease in the number of carelessly discarded needles and syringes in public places where previously there were many.

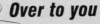

Over to you

Next time you take part in an intervention to promote a change in behaviour, such as the introduction of healthy snacks in a school, observe how people behave during the initiative. How successful was the initiative? Would you have modified the initiative in any way?

Reflection

Reflection lends itself to process evaluation. Practitioners examine what was achieved and how it was achieved. They identify aspects of the initiative that worked well or could be improved. They identify what was learned through the process and what could be changed next time. Reflection can be used with other types of evaluation.

Key points Top tips

- Evaluation of public health interventions is complex
- Evaluation is often divided into outcome evaluation and process evaluation
- Evaluation can involve quantitative data, qualitative data or both
- Think carefully about the intervention and choose the most appropriate evaluation method that will give accurate and valid conclusions

Evaluating different approaches to health promotion

The approach of the health promotion activity will influence the method of evaluation. Ewles and Simnett (2003) identify five major categories of approach: medical, behaviour change, educational, radical or social change, and empowerment. Each of these approaches has a different type of outcome or goal. If we regard evaluation as determination of effectiveness through assessing the extent to which predetermined goals have been met, the evaluation method will depend on the approach to health promotion.

A medical approach to health promotion includes interventions that depend on medical knowledge, such as immunisation campaigns and screening programmes. Here the goals are related to the size of the target population that receives the intervention and, in screening programmes, the number of people whose condition is detected early enough to treat it. A behaviour change approach aims to persuade individuals to change some health-damaging aspect of their behaviour, such as too much alcohol or too little physical exercise. The goals are directly related to the desired change in behaviour and can be measured by the numbers of people who have made that change.

An educational approach aims to develop service users' knowledge and understanding of their health experiences in the hope that their attitude and then their behaviour will change in line with their new understanding. Tones and Tilford (1994) argue that besides giving them information, education empowers people and promotes their ability to process new knowledge and use it to inform decisions and actions. The goals of this approach relate to the extent to which people are informed about a particular health issue and the extent to which they can articulate a reasoned approach to decisions about that issue.

A radical or social change approach aims to 'make the healthier option the easier option' (Department of Health 1999) by changing factors in a person's environment so that healthy options are made more accessible or more possible. The goals of this approach are related to policy, structural and environmental changes and subsequent changes in behaviour. An empowerment or community development approach aims to facilitate participants in the self-directed identification of health needs and the design and implementation of actions to address those needs. The goals relate to the extent to which participants engage in the process and succeed in taking planned actions.

Evidence base

Taylor, M., Purdis, D., Wilson, M. and Wilde, P. (2005) *Evaluating Community Projects: A Practical Guide*. Joseph Rowntree Foundation, York. Download it at the Foundation's website.

Table 8.1 summarises the five approaches to health promotion, the types of intervention they use and the evaluation methods to consider.

Table 8.1 Five approaches to health promotion

Approach	Type of intervention	Evaluation method
Medical	Screening programme	Statistical data collection of numbers screened and numbers of successful early interventions
Behaviour change	Media campaign aimed at stopping smoking	Statistical data collection of incidence of smoking behaviour and trends
Educational	Classes that teach young parents to cook on a budget and how to use more fruit and vegetables in the family diet	Questionnaire to establish what has been learned and what action is intended. Follow-up to ascertain what actions have been taken
Radical or social change	Campaigns to persuade the local education authority to introduce a policy that gives access to healthy drinks and snacks during lesson breaks	Introduction of new policy. Statistical data on uptake of healthy snacks in schools
Empowerment or community development	Working with groups of local mothers to identify the need for improved children's play facilities and enable them to lobby the local authority so they get them	Success in lobbying for change. Process evaluation questionnaire to measure the mothers' degree of empowerment or enablement

When evaluating public health interventions it can be difficult to establish how much of any change was produced by the intervention (Green and South 2006). The case study below is a good illustration.

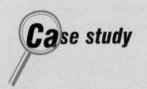

Case study

Jane campaigns on influenza

Jane leads a team of six part-time practice nurses at a large and busy general practice in a seaside town. A large proportion of its registered patients are older people as the town is a popular retirement destination. Last year the practice had difficulty dealing with many home visits or arranging hospital care for older people who fell ill during a localised influenza epidemic and there were more deaths than expected. This year Jane was asked to maximise the uptake of influenza vaccine among the eligible population. She and her team tried to encourage uptake using posters, personal invitations, opportunistic interventions and other strategies.

To evaluate the success of her campaign, Jane had all vaccinations properly recorded on the practice's computer system. Her data analysis showed that 79 per cent of eligible patients over 65 received their vaccination this year compared with 73 per cent; the national average for last year was 74 per cent. Jane's data showed many fewer hospital admissions and fewer influenza-related deaths than the same time last year. The GPs and the practice manager were pleased with these results and promised to give her resources to run a similar campaign next year.

- Do you think that Jane's campaign was a success?
- What other explanation could there be for the fall in influenza-related hospital admissions and deaths?
- What other types of data could Jane have collected to support her evaluation?

Was Jane's campaign successful? The answer partly depends on what she was trying to achieve. She was asked to increase the uptake of the influenza vaccine among the practice population, so we might assume that the ultimate aim was to reduce morbidity and mortality from influenza. On first consideration the data suggests that Jane's campaign successfully encouraged more people to come to the surgery for their influenza vaccination and this reduced the number of hospital admissions and deaths related to influenza. But closer consideration shows that several factors might have contributed to this outcome. For example, local people may also be aware of the effects of last year's epidemic and this alone may have influenced many more people to get vaccinated. National publicity and media messages encouraging people to have a flu vaccination may have had a greater impact than previously.

Even if Jane could ascertain that her campaign encouraged a greater uptake of vaccinations, she could not be certain that this, by itself, had led to fewer hospital admissions and deaths. There may have been a less virulent strain of influenza this year or there may have been more people nursed at home by community nursing services. That is why several evaluation methods may be needed to obtain more concrete evidence that a particular intervention has been effective. Besides collecting statistics, Jane could have interviewed people who attended for vaccination and asked them what influenced their decision to attend. She could have consulted the practice's computer to find out how many consultations might have been related to the symptoms of influenza. She could have asked the community nursing team how many cases of influenza had been nursed at home this year.

A medical approach evaluated by collecting and analysing statistical data may initially seem far more robust than, say, a community development approach, but have a look at the case study below.

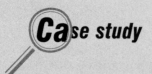

Sarah tackles child road accidents

Sarah is a school nurse. She is based in a large, new children's centre on a housing estate in the suburbs of a large city in central England. She has worked in the area for three years and produced family needs assessments and family health promotion initiatives. Through analysing her records for those three years, Sarah spotted a steady rise in the number of notifications from the local A & E department for children injured in road accidents or while playing outside in the street. This made her concerned, and when several parents made informal comments about children injured in road accidents, she began to think that residents were also concerned. She set up an open meeting at the children's centre and invited residents to come and discuss the issue. Her aim was to facilitate local residents in expressing their concerns and to support them in identifying possible solutions.

A small number of parents came to the meeting. They were hesitant at first but they grew quite animated. Sarah arranged another meeting and many more people came. The parents at the first meeting had spread the word. The people at the second meeting decided to call themselves a community action group and to have more meetings to discuss how they could improve the estate's play facilities for children and

Continued

young people. They proposed that a small play area on some unused land near the centre of the estate would help encourage children away from football on the streets, but they wanted support from the local authority. Sarah helped the group contact a local authority representative and they invited him to speak at their next meeting. After that, the group met regularly without Sarah's involvement and eventually persuaded the local authority to create a play area on the estate.

- Do you think that Sarah's intervention was effective?
- Suggest the most appropriate methods to evaluate Sarah's intervention.

Sarah's intervention was introduced as a community development initiative. A community development initiative has outcome goals and process goals. The term 'community development' implies some positive change in a community and the people who belong to it. Sarah arranged a meeting as she was concerned about the rising number of children who arrived at A & E because they were injured in the streets. One of the outcome goals for Sarah's intervention could be to reduce the number of children who arrive at A & E because they are injured in the streets. This could be evaluated by a quantitative analysis of referral data, similar to Sarah's analysis before she arranged the meeting. She could simply count the number of attendances and compare the rate of attendance before and after her intervention. Before claiming that her intervention had reduced the numbers, she would need to account for other factors that may have had an effect. Indeed the group members may feel strongly that the outcome was directly attributable to their own efforts and nothing to do with Sarah's involvement.

This leads us to consider another of Sarah's goals – to empower or enable the residents to identify their own problems then suggest and pursue their own solutions. This is an outcome goal and a process goal that can be evaluated by finding out whether the members of the group felt more able to solve their problems after Sarah's meeting than before Sarah's meeting. It could be evaluated using questionnaires or interviews on the residents' feelings about the way Sarah had intervened and the outcomes of her intervention.

So was Sarah's intervention effective? As always, the answer depends on knowing Sarah's goals. One of her goals may have been to reduce the number of accidents to children in the street. The case study does not contain enough information to determine this. It would require data to be analysed over time. Another of Sarah's goals may have been to engage and enable local residents to identify and tackle their own concerns. Here it seems that Sarah did have some success. The great advantage of achieving this goal is that the residents will probably be able to tackle some of their other concerns without further intervention from Sarah or another public health practitioner. Sarah's intervention could help the residents achieve many more goals but they are yet to be identified.

Evidence base

Taylor, M., Purdis, D., Wilson, M. and Wilde, P. (2005) *Evaluating Community Projects: A Practical Guide*. Joseph Rowntree Foundation, York. Download it at the Foundation's website.

The case study on page 147 was about a population and the one on page 148 was about a community. The next case study is about a person and uses an educational approach.

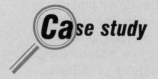

Case study

Alison explains breastfeeding

Alison is a newly qualified midwife. She has a small caseload in a thriving market town, home to the families of many young professionals who commute to jobs in the city. This morning she received a telephone call from Anne, a young mother who wants some help to decide whether she should continue to breastfeed or start to bottle-feed her 6-day-old baby. Alison is working to increase the duration of breastfeeding among her caseload and sees this as an opportunity for some one-to-one health education.

- Suggest some realistic goals for Alison's health education session with Anne.
- What information would she need to collect to evaluate her session?
- How should she obtain this information?

Among Alison's goals, it might be expected that she hoped to provide information for Anne and to enable her to use the information to help with decision making. This could be evaluated through informal feedback from Anne relating to whether she feels better informed and more able to make an appropriate decision. One problem with educational outcomes such as these is that they do not specify an outcome which is clearly identifiable as contributing to the achievement of specified public health targets. It may be that Anne accepts all the information on the advantages and disadvantages of breastfeeding and bottle-feeding and decides to bottle-feed her baby. But it is likely that Alison is also keen to promote the continuation of breastfeeding in this case and therefore contributes to achieving her goal for her caseload.

Evaluation of this type of outcome relates to Anne's decision and her ability to make a decision that is satisfactory and appropriate for her own priorities. As in the earlier case studies, evaluation must be clearly related to the goals. In this case, Alison may achieve the educational outcomes she has set, but to achieve her goal on breastfeeding duration, perhaps it might have been more appropriate for Alison to adopt a behaviour change approach. This raises the idea that each approach implies a different type of goal, and these goals may not be accorded equal value by all concerned. In this case, policy makers and performance managers in Alison's authority may not see education and empowerment as legitimate outcomes.

Conclusion

To evaluate a public health intervention, you must clearly articulate its goals. Even then, the evaluation may be difficult and contentious. Yet it is very difficult to defend public health interventions that have not been evaluated; decision makers may regard them as worthless or a waste of professional time. As evaluation becomes more embedded in public health practice, an evidence base will develop and public health approaches will become better established and more valued as meaningful and effective interventions.

All public health practitioners can contribute by choosing appropriate evaluation methods when they plan their interventions and by collecting adequate data to do the analysis. Proper evaluation will considerably enhance public health practice by making it more valuable and more effective. The process of evaluating public health interventions can be summarised in four steps based on advice from *Making It Happen: A Guide to Mental Health Promotion* (Department of Health 2001b):

1. Set aims and objectives for the intervention so the elements to be evaluated are identified at the start of the process.

2. Identify evaluation indicators so the people involved in the evaluation know what data to collect and in what format.

3. Choose an evaluation method that suits the type of intervention plus its aims and objectives.

4. Explain the evaluation method to all participants so they know what to do during the evaluation process.

Rapid recap

Check your progress so far by working through each of the following questions.

1. What is outcome evaluation?
2. What is process evaluation?
3. What are the purposes of evaluation?
4. List five approaches that can be used for evaluation.
5. Why is goal setting so important for evaluation?

If you have difficulty with more than one of the questions, read through the section again to refresh your understanding before moving on.

References

Aggleton, P. and Chalmers, H. (1986) *Nursing Models and the Nursing Process*. Macmillan, Basingstoke, Hants.

Bowling, A. (2002) *Research Methods in Health*, 2nd edn. Open University Press, Maidenhead, Berks.

Craig, P. and Smith, N. (1998) Health visiting and public health: back to our roots or a new branch. *Health and Social Care in the Community*, **6**(3), 172–180.

Department of Health (1999) *Saving Lives: Our Healthier Nation*. HMSO, London.

Department of Health (2001a) *A Research Development Strategy for Public Health*. HMSO, London.

Department of Health (2001b) *Making It Happen: A Guide to Mental Health Promotion*. HMSO, London, www.dh.gov.uk, accessed 27 July 2007.

Elkan, R., Mitch, B. and Robinson, J. (2000) Evidence-based practice and health visiting: the need for theoretical underpinnings for evaluation. *Journal of Advanced Nursing*, **31**(6), 1316–1323.

Ewles, L. and Simnett, I. (1999) *Promoting Health*, 4th edn. Baillière Tindall, Edinburgh.

Ewles, L. and Simnett, I. (2003) *Promoting Health*, 5th edn. Baillière Tindall, London.

General Nursing Council for England and Wales (1977) *Training Syllabus Register of Nurses*. GNC, London.

Glasgow, R., Vogt, T. and Boles, S. (1999) Evaluating the public health impact of health promotion interventions: the RE-AIM framework. *American Journal of Public Health*, **89**(9), 1322–1327.

Green, J. and South, J. (2006) *Evaluation*. Open University Press, Maidenhead, Berks.

Naidoo, J. and Wills, J. (2000) *Health Promotion: Foundations for Practice*. Ballière Tindall, London.

Neary, M. (2000) *Teaching, Assessing and Evaluation for Clinical Competence: A Practical Guide for Practitioners and Teachers*. Stanley Thornes, Cheltenham, Glos.

Plews, C., Billingham, K. and Rowe, A. (2000) Public health nursing: barriers and opportunities. *Health and Social Care in the Community*, **8**(2), 138–146.

Polit, D. and Hungler, B. (1993) *Nursing Research Methods: Appraisal and Utilization*. Lippincott, Philadelphia PA.

Taylor, M., Purdis, D., Wilson, M. and Wilde, P. (2005) *Evaluating Community Projects: A Practical Guide*. Joseph Rowntree Foundation, York.

Tones, K. and Green, J. (2004) *Health Promotion, Planning and Strategies*. Sage, London.

Tones, K. and Tilford, S. (1994) *Health Education: Effectiveness, Efficiency and Equity* Chapman & Hall, London.

Yura, H. and Walsh, M. B. (1967) *The Nursing Process*. Appleton Century Crofts, New York.

9
Leading public health developments

Scott Harrison and Liz Berry

Learning outcomes

By the end of this chapter you should be able to:

★ Understand the broader role of public health nursing globally and locally

★ Identify the steps required to successfully lead public health initiatives

★ Define effective leadership in public health practice

★ Consider the use of a practice development framework in developing public health practice.

Introduction

This chapter shows how the principles of public health can be applied in public health nursing – nurses registered on Part 3 of the NMC register or similar. It shares the experiences of public health nurses from a variety of situations in the UK and abroad. The chapter is written entirely from the perspective of public health nurses working in practice.

Seven steps to successful practice

Whatever the initiative or approach, we have found that seven essential steps will ensure the success of public health nursing initiatives.

Step 1 Engage people

Engage people from a variety of situations, occupations, cultures and communities. A key skill is the ability to read situations and people, sometimes quite quickly, and decide how to deliver your message in the most acceptable and meaningful way. This requires an advanced state of emotional intelligence (EI) – core abilities concerned with understanding how and why we feel and behave as we do, particularly in relation to others (Bar-On and Parker 2000). These abilities are essential currency in Goleman's conceptualisation of EI (Goleman 1995, 1998), which is perhaps most usefully defined as 'the ability to monitor one's own and other's emotions, to discriminate among them and to use the information to guide one's thinking and actions' (Salovey and Mayer 1990, p.189).

If public health nursing is to be truly emancipatory and ameliorating, EI is essential in ensuring that patients' or clients' holistic needs are addressed and that they are helped to manage not only their physical health, but also to gain greater insight into and management of their emotional world (McQueen 2004). Some people may not be receptive to public health messages because they lack trust in mainstream services, often because these services are perceived as patronising or stigmatising. The effective public health nurse has to be able to understand and accept this, yet, still find a way to re-engage the person or group. Equally important is the ability to manage situations where no progress is currently possible and to develop strategies that allow the practitioner to cope with and manage this frustration while still being helpful to the client.

Step 2 Be a community leader

The skills that public health nurses develop in their daily work with individuals, groups and larger communities are often centred on negotiating partnerships and constructing collaborative initiatives that build on the strengths of the communities they serve. As a result, they are ideally positioned to manage the delivery of a wide variety of services within a restructured system that allocates more realistic resources to wellness initiatives. Practically this means raising your profile and being prepared to challenge boundaries and become involved in activities that might be outside your comfort zone or perceived responsibility, such as a public health nurse lobbying to be included on the board of a local homeless hostel committee, or bringing together community leaders to form a health action group. It's about being prepared to take a lead and take some risks. Nurses too often think they are not influential enough to take on leadership roles, but in public health this could not be further from the truth. Expert understanding of the principles of public health makes public health nurses natural community leaders.

Step 3 Be a service leader

Constant engagement in community activities requires negotiation and brokerage skills that make public health nurses highly effective members and often leaders of interdisciplinary and inter-agency teams. The art of successful networking is a key public health skill that should not be underestimated. An understanding of the wider determinants of health naturally calls for inter-agency working to ensure that joined-up solutions are formed for public health issues with multiple factors. As experts in community and public health, we can readily provide leadership to teams of community practitioners such as peer health educators, outreach workers, community involvement officers and general practitioners. Public health nurses should embrace the opportunity to lead teams which act as community resource networks, working with communities to identify and solve their shared health issues.

Public health nurse

We are a group of public health nurses in a PCT in north-west England. We have developed partnerships with social service training departments to ensure that lay carers are equipped to promote health and support self-care for the people they work with. This is an effective partnership between care agency managers, educators, carers and public health nurses and raises awareness of health needs.

Step 4 Deliver care in a community-based framework

Community-based services should be driven by the needs and resources of the community and its neighbourhoods. Public health nurses are in the ideal position to assess communities on a daily basis as part of their work with individuals, families and groups in schools, neighbourhoods, workplaces and homes. Be aware of the models that exist to support your work and use them to plan and deliver public health strategies. Traditional health-care models tend to rely on three core predictive variables:

- genetic predisposition
- environmental factors
- health behaviours.

When measuring health, professionals often rely on morbidities and the frequency of health-care contact (Chapter 5). This approach rarely includes functional health – the ability of the person to manage in their environment and successfully perform their daily activities. For example, a person with asthma may be measured by health professionals as having improved peak flow, but what about their ability to exercise, to laugh with friends without coughing, walk around the shopping mall without having to use their medication several times? Functional health is what matters to the person, not information that helps health professionals measure their physical or emotional health. Health information is essential but it should be used as part of a more comprehensive assessment.

To provide a more meaningful model for public health practice, researchers working in the US developed the family–community health promotion (FCHP) model (Mendoza and Fuentes-Afflick 1999). They were seeking to understand the epidemiological paradox of immigrant children living in poverty who demonstrated positive health outcomes. The FCHP model retains the three core predictive variables of traditional models but adds several new ones. It focuses more closely on the family–community axis than on the genetic–behaviour axis. A major supposition of the model is that, if a community promotes beneficial health behaviours among its members, these lessons become part of the community's signifying practices. This can include dietary preference, alcohol use and core health values. If public health nurses can work with the community to influence health behaviours, these will be passed down in the dynamic process of community history and signifying practices.

> ### Over to you
>
> Read Mendoza, F. S. and Fuentes-Afflick, E. (1999) Latino children's health and the family–community health promotion model, *Western Journal of Medicine,* **170**, 85–92. Concentrate on what the authors say about the 'silver bullet' approach of modern medicine and whether this is effective in public health.

Step 5 Make links with community resource networks

There is a growing emphasis on health in communities. Many previously disadvantaged groups and neglected neighbourhoods are waking up to the reality that health is everybody's business. To ensure the future quality of health information and support available to communities, public health nurses must be a central and accessible point for health information and support. Public health nurses should learn about what is happening in their community and what services are available already. This reduces the risk of duplicating effort and helps you tap into the community's skills and resources. It may include finding out what local businesses in the area are interested in community development, such as by contacting a local supermarket to source free or cheap food to support a healthy-eating group for new parents or to offer free fruit at community clinics.

Step 6 Make links with regional, national and international colleagues

Public health nurses need to link to colleagues and initiatives beyond their local boundaries. Do Once and Share, from NHS Connecting for Health in the UK, is pioneering national approaches to common health issues so it can cut duplication in spending and human effort. Broad links through practice development units, interest groups and international web communities are essential for developing a common direction and common strategies. Sharing information on evidence-based practice is as essential as sharing information on trends in emerging communicable diseases, epidemiological issues, community development, sexual health and the impact of government policy on health.

> ### Over to you
>
> Identify a successful piece of work you have been involved in. List ways that you could share this success with other public health practitioners. Write down the steps to turn a local project into a national initiative. Go to the Connecting for Health website for some help.

Step 7 Give priority to high-risk populations

Practical application covers all the principles of public health nursing, so it is often the largest challenge you will face. For maximum effectiveness, illness prevention strategies and campaigns to improve well-being should be targeted to identify and intervene with people and groups who are at high risk of injury or illness. Although health promotion is relevant to everyone and to all communities, regardless of risk status, the reality of scarce resources means it may be most effective to target health promotion strategies at populations with the poorest health status. This aspect of public health nursing is often the most challenging.

Working with high-risk groups often lacks engagement from patients and policy makers, so public health nurses must use their strong backbone. Often the information you are delivering is not what people want to hear about their life or their policy making. Marginalised communities are sensitive and challenging environments, but big changes can be made with perseverance and determination. The next section gives some examples to demonstrate how public health nurses have accepted these challenges and overcome significant barriers.

Recap of the seven steps to success:

1. Engage people.
2. Be a community leader.
3. Be a service leader.
4. Deliver care in a community-based framework.
5. Make links with community resource networks.
6. Make links with regional, national and international colleagues.
7. Give priority to high-risk populations.

⚿ Keywords

Learning disability
A disability that significantly reduces a person's ability to understand new information, to learn new skills (impaired intelligence) with a reduced ability to cope independently (impaired social function) that started before adulthood and has a lasting effect on a person's development (Department of Health 2001)

Public health developments

Learning disabilities

The health of people with a **learning disability** has long been an area of concern. Change has been slow despite a range of reports and policy recommendations (Department of Health 1999; Mencap 2004). People

○━┱ *Keywords*

Social communication disorder

A disorder classified as a neurodevelopmental disorder that manifests itself in markedly abnormal social interaction, communication ability, patterns of interests, and patterns of behaviour (Strock 2004). Also called autism

with learning disabilities have seen a gradual increase in life expectancy but their mortality rates indicate significantly increased risk of early death compared to the general population, particularly for patients with Down's syndrome and profound and multiple learning disabilities (PMLD). When they are ill, people with learning disabilities and **social communication disorders** visit their GP with a similar frequency as the general population, but they are much less likely to receive regular health checks or to access health promotion and health improvement activities (Mencap 2004).

> ## Over to you
>
> Go to the Mencap website and read the report 'Treat Me Right' about the health needs and health-care experiences of people with learning disabilities.

Access All Areas, Warrington, UK

Description

Access All Areas is a programme for delivering primary health care that has its roots firmly in the principles of social justice and public health (Harrison and Berry 2006). By incorporating the specialist input of dedicated learning disability services with mainstream primary care services, it makes a joint effort to challenge exclusion and address the agenda of *Valuing People* (Department of Health 2001). The service facilitates illness-related care, improves health and well-being, and addresses the causes of ill health for people with learning disabilities.

Goals and objectives

In partnership with specialist services and service users, Access All Areas is a comprehensive programme using a public health model of health care where people with learning disabilities are supported to have their health assessed, make healthy choices and, often for the first time, are given information in accessible formats to support those choices. The focus of Access All Areas is to facilitate access to mainstream primary care services, avoiding two-tier systems of health care that research shows to be ineffective and often of poor quality. It fully embraces the principle of full partnership working with patients. The service aims to case-manage patients with long-term conditions and to develop programmes which support wellness in this marginalised group.

Background

People with a learning disability have spent decades being excluded from mainstream society and remain almost invisible in our communities, workplaces and in family life. As a result, the health of people with a learning disability is significantly poorer than the health of the general population (Thornton 1999). Despite the many reports and policy recommendations about how to improve the situation, little has been done to address the social exclusion of this group, and their health and well-being continue to decline (Department of Health 1998). In a joint effort to challenge exclusion and address the agenda of *Valuing People*, Warrington PCT and 5 Boroughs Partnership NHS Trust joined forces at a practical level – two public health nurses have developed a comprehensive programme of socially inclusive health care aimed at engaging people with learning disabilities more fully in their health care and their choices in leading healthy lives.

Programme overview

All general practices in the PCT have developed a register of patients with learning disabilities with support from the Access All Areas team. Each patient identified by the project is considered individually and their communication and other needs are identified wherever possible in a team approach with community learning disability nurses and specialist speech and language therapists. Nursing staff based in primary care are encouraged and assisted to assess the current health status of each patient using a standardised health needs assessment (HNA) tool developed by the project workers. This HNA tool includes the significant health issues of people with learning disabilities. For patients with existing complex health needs, a community matron is employed for comprehensive HNA and clinical case management (Department of Health 2005). An essential part of the project has been to let patients or clients see and own their health information and health history.

The project has implemented the use of patient-held health profiles to ensure that patients or clients have ownership of personal information and are included in their care. These profiles are very similar to the personal child health record (PCHR) in that they contain the patient's main health information and provide an active record for staff to make notes in. A health action plan is contained in the profile to help patients and carers identify health needs, formulate a simple plan to meet those needs, and identify who in the patient's life can support the plan. The core of this process is providing patients with choices about their health and lifestyle and facilitating healthy choices where possible. The comprehensive joint training programme offered to primary care staff and social carers includes the main areas of concern: roles, responsibilities, the core difficulties of learning disabilities, the problems of accessing health care and some potential solutions.

How it demonstrates the key activities of public health

- **Engage people** – Access All Areas jointly funded a health inequalities project manager with the borough council to establish better anticipatory care and ensure that people with learning disabilities have equal access to leisure, prevention services, health promotion, healthy eating and health-enhancing activities. It works with advocacy groups to design and deliver the programme.

- **Be community leaders** – Access All Areas has a partnership with the borough council joint training partnership to ensure that all social care staff employed in local social care agencies have health awareness and health promotion education as part of their induction and ongoing development.

- **Be service leaders** – public health nurses give clinical leadership on the project; they establish and chair forums for service users and key stakeholders.

- **Deliver care in a community-based framework** – a 12-week health awareness raising project (HARP) raises the self-awareness of people with learning disabilities and helps them make healthy choices and improve their health in partnership with existing health promotion services and based on the principles of functional health.

- **Make links with community resource networks** – a community food initiative helps people with learning disabilities grow, sell and cook their own fresh fruit and vegetables.

- **Make wider links** – Access All Areas developed its anticipatory care calendar with the national cancer inequalities network and the strategic health authority. This makes daily assessments of people with severe learning disabilities and tracks changes in their health. In partnership, Access All Areas is developing a national care pathway for health action planning.

- **Give priority to high-risk populations** – the service was based on national evidence and delivered to a community known to be at risk of poor health.

Keywords

Homelessness

According to the UK Housing Act 1996, a person is homeless if they have no accommodation that they are entitled to occupy or they have accommodation but it is not reasonable for them to continue occupying it. There are wider definitions of 'rough sleeping' and 'sofa-surfing' but the legal definition considers the right to a home, not the circumstances in which someone lacks a home

Homelessness, refugees and people seeking asylum

Homelessness and asylum have recently emerged as prime focuses of UK social policy in the broader context of social exclusion (Social Exclusion Unit 2004). This is a response to real and identifiable needs, particularly the needs of increasing numbers of homeless people and asylum applicants plus broader trends and issues. Biomedical theories that often guide the work of the health services do not explain the health impact of these social issues (Young 2006), which often have negative health consequences. Homelessness has significant consequences for the homeless person and the wider community. Homeless people and asylum applicants experience poorer levels of general physical and mental health than the general population and substantial evidence from around the world documents multiple morbidity. Despite this, homeless people often have problems obtaining suitable health care (Wright and Tompkins 2006).

Downtown Community Health Centre, Vancouver, Canada

Description

The Downtown Community Health Centre (DCHC) model encompasses an approach that addresses the physical, spiritual or traditional, mental and emotional needs of disadvantaged people with complex social and health-care needs, many of whom are from First Nations communities, intravenous drug users, sex workers or homeless (Benoit *et al.* 2003).

Goals and objectives

The Positive Outlook programme was established in 1993 to provide care treatment and support services to all people living with HIV/ Aids, focusing on the need to improve access to care for First Nations people. The programme received extra funding in 1997 to expand care treatment and support services.

Background

Most of the clients accessing the programme live on Vancouver's Downtown Eastside. This is one of Canada's poorest urban neighbourhoods and is characterised by unemployment, crime, mental illness, prostitution and inadequate housing. The community's harsh social environment and crippling poverty perpetuate the serious health consequences facing its residents. Traditional service delivery models are often ineffectual for this population. DCHC has set up an integrated, innovative, comprehensive health-care model to improve clients' acceptance of services and compliance with treatment regimes.

Programme overview

The primary mandate is to provide treatment services to vulnerable clients. The model bridges the gap between hospital, community and the myriad specialised services in Vancouver's Downtown Eastside. Respect for First Nations cultures forms a basic tenet of the programme. Flexible approaches recognise the complexity of needs and the individual situation of each client. Components include daily drop-in, food bank, meals, crisis intervention, legal advocacy, counselling, prevention education, maximally assisted medication therapy, and on-site access to physicians, nurses, social workers, addiction counsellors and outreach workers. Staff collaborate in and out of the programme and work with clients wherever needed, including hospital. Strong partnerships were formed with all existing Aids organisations plus ongoing consultation and involvement in discharge planning with St Paul's Hospital.

How it demonstrates the key activities of public health

- **Engage people** – DCHC is based in the community it serves and includes service users consistently. It recognises the difficulties experienced by marginalised groups in accessing and engaging with services and the difficulties experienced by mainstream services in delivering care to this community. Its service aims to address these difficulties.

- **Be community leaders** – DCHC coordinates a community-based approach that engages multiple agencies in delivering responsive, active and preventive services.
- **Be service leaders** – public health nurses give clinical leadership on how to engage highly vulnerable individuals that are hard to reach. They have a high profile in DCHC.
- **Deliver care in a community-based framework** – DCHC's care focuses on improving functional health and addressing the wider determinants of poor health. DCHC recognises the complex lives of the people it serves and takes a coordinated approach to reduce harm and improve engagement with treatment.
- **Make links with community resource networks** – DCHC uses all existing preventive and supportive services and works in partnership with multiple resource networks to ensure that patients are directed to the most appropriate support.
- **Make wider links** – DCHC has a high profile in Canada and other countries as it provides ground-breaking services, including the first legal supervised injection site for intravenous drug users.
- **Give priority to high-risk populations** – the service is based on evidence and local experience of a community in Downtown Eastside known to be at risk of poor health and major social problems.

People and communities outside mainstream services

Social exclusion relates to the disenfranchisement or alienation experienced by some people in society. It is often related to a person's class, education, ethnicity, gender, living standards or lifestyle. Anyone who deviates in any perceived way from the norm of a population can become subject to overt or more pervasive forms of social exclusion. The problems are linked and become mutually reinforcing, creating a vicious cycle in people's lives. As the world changes at an ever faster pace, it throws up increasing challenges to social life. Public health nurses need to prepare to meet these challenges and find ways to help communities meet them (Department of Health 2004).

The sociologist Manuel Castells has studied cities, networks and global development. He has observed the rapidly increasing growth of a 'fourth world' – black holes of social exclusion cut off from the flow of wealth and information in the global economy and as likely to appear in a Western city as in sub-Saharan Africa (Castells 2000). Because they are disconnected from the rest of the world, these places are powerless and unable to change. Some neighbourhoods in UK cities and towns experience increasing levels of crime, poor health and poverty that cause people and communities to become disenfranchised. According to the Social Exclusion Unit (2004), this has led governments to begin adopting policies which:

- tackle key economic causes of social exclusion, such as unemployment and poverty, particularly child and pensioner poverty
- promote equal opportunities for all
- support communities, particularly in deprived areas
- reintegrate some of those who have experienced more extreme forms of social exclusion, like rough sleeping
- improve access to advice and services.

> **Over to you**
>
> Go to the Cabinet Office's website and read the report on social exclusion. This will help you understand social exclusion and policy decisions on social exclusion.

Multiple and Complex Needs Initiative, Victoria, Australia

Description

Since January 2002 the Department of Human Services in Victoria, Australia, has run a project to develop and implement strategies for people with multiple and complex needs. These people may become involved with a wide range of services but without clear case management and funding responsibility or they may be referred from service to service as they do not meet legislative requirements for eligibility. Services may include mental health, disability, child protection, juvenile justice, drug treatment, housing and support programmes, and care of the aged. The new service response targets people aged 16 and older with multiple and complex needs. It is centred on a time-limited specialist intervention that aims to stabilise housing, health, social connection and safety issues; pursue planned and consistent therapeutic goals for each individual; and provide a platform for long-term engagement in the service system (Department of Human Services 2007).

Goals and objectives

- To provide an individualised and tailored service response to assist in managing people's complex needs.
- To identify, quantify and develop a comprehensive profile of the types of people with complex needs – the target group – and the costs and resources associated with service provision to these people.
- To identify strengths and weaknesses of current legislative frameworks that define the provision of services to the target group.
- To identify strengths and weaknesses of policy frameworks and service responses plus any gaps in services.

- To identify examples of best practice, including anecdotal examples, plus local and international evidence-based research on service provision.
- To develop a service framework and strategic plan for improving responses to the target group, taking into account current resource use, potential resource demands and future workforce requirements.
- To define appropriate service responses and propose how resources can be reallocated to provide them.
- To recommend how service solutions may be supported by legislative change.

Background

Over the past few years, concerns have been raised about the difficulty of providing services to a group of people who have multiple and complex needs. These concerns have been raised by service providers, clinicians, carers, the Office of the Public Advocate, the police, magistrates and others. The group of people often considered to have complex needs includes people who may experience various combinations of mental illness, intellectual disability, acquired brain injury, physical disability, behavioural difficulties, social isolation, family dysfunction, and drug or alcohol misuse. They are often unable to sustain appropriate accommodation or require a level of support that the current service designs do not readily allow. Services often cannot maintain long-term involvement with people who have extremely difficult behaviours. Many of these people are homeless or at risk of homelessness.

How it demonstrates the key activities of public health

- **Engage people** – the service is aimed at a hard-to-reach population who find it difficult to engage with services for a variety of reasons. It aims to engage all partners in health and social care who have previously been unable or unwilling to engage with this hard-to-reach population.
- **Be community leaders** – the service has mobilised community activity to form a coherent service that leads by example and demonstrates to patients that coordinated support is achievable.
- **Be service leaders** – the service uses a multiple and complex needs panel to assess referrals, determine eligibility and appoint a case coordinator, release brokerage funds and assess ongoing care plans.
- **Deliver care in a community-based framework** – the service works closely with the person being helped and with local service providers to strengthen the capacity of the service system to provide support to the person in their own community and improve functional health and well-being.

- **Make links with community resource networks** – the service uses a multidisciplinary approach to assess needs then plan and deliver care. It expects patients to be returned to mainstream community services as soon as possible. This ensures a successful transition of care plan coordination from the specialist team to a local service provider within the period of the care plan.
- **Make wider links** – regional coordinators advise on the referral process and eligibility criteria so the service provides a single point of access for referrals.
- **Give priority to high-risk populations** – the service provides intensive case management support to people who do not have an identified care plan coordinator. Strict referral criteria ensure the service supports the people most in need and prevents it from being diluted.

Over to you

Thinking globally, acting locally! Having read the information on social exclusion and vulnerable communities, prepare a plan that identifies which aspects of social exclusion are prevalent in your area and that identifies one key activity you could do to address meaningful issues in your community. Say how this plan might be supported by the people who commission health care in your area.

Making it happen

Public health practitioners must be able to develop and promote services that begin to unpick the multiple factors of social exclusion and that help people develop skills and access the services to improve and maintain their health. Sometimes this can feel totally overwhelming, but a good starting point is to discover which aspects of social exclusion are particularly prevalent in your own geographical area. For some, this may mean helping rural farming communities to address mental health and coping skills (Chapter 4); for others it may be engaging communities on run-down estates with multiple disadvantages. We hope we have provided you with a flavour of what can be achieved in practice.

Public health and practice development

This section looks at practice development by an integrated public health team working in north-west England (Kiddy 2007). This inner-city public health team set up a practice development unit (PDU) that used an approach to practice development pioneered by the Centre for the Development of Policy and Practice (Department of Health 2003). Figure 9.1 shows a Venn diagram where practice development is the intersection of creativity and innovation, quality improvement and evidence base.

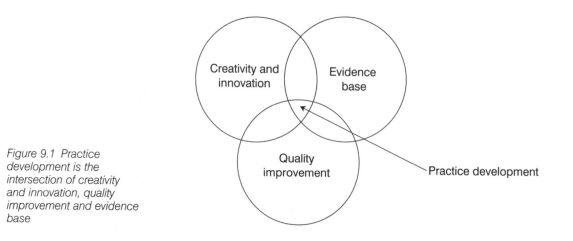

Figure 9.1 Practice development is the intersection of creativity and innovation, quality improvement and evidence base

Practice development

The 15 criteria in Box 9.1 form a framework for practice development (Totterdell 2004). Each criterion, supported by a body of evidence, forms a strand of the rope that links effective practice development, in this case public health development, with improved outcomes for patients, clients or communities.

Box 9.1

Practice development framework

1. The PDU has a clear and defined client focus, which is reflected in the membership of the team
2. The team has chosen the accreditation approach itself
3. The team has a shared vision for the PDU
4. An approach to leadership is identified which will facilitate the team in sustainable development, evaluation and dissemination of its work
5. The PDU has an explicit framework for developing best practice, which incorporates devolved decision making, staff and patient empowerment, and partnership working
6. Each member of the team is proactively involved in self-development clearly related to patient or client need
7. The PDU's development plan identifies the resources required
8. The PDU's development plan includes the process for disseminating evaluated practices within the organisation and externally
9. The team has a reciprocal partnership with a centre for education to support the development of clinical practice and theory
10. The team develops a rigorous evidence-based approach to practice

Continued

11. The team is actively engaged in reflection and learning from practice experience
12. The team exhibits tangible evidence of creativity and innovation in relation to patient or client issues
13. Developments within the unit are evaluated and reviewed in terms of their impact on the patient or client organisation, and staff advise the board
14. The team acts as an agent of change in the organisation, regionally and nationally
15. The team has a steering group to help focus and coordinate the strategic direction of the PDU

Evidence base

Read this literature review: McCormack, B., Wright, J., Dewar, B., Harvey, G. and Ballantine, K. (2007) A realist synthesis of evidence relating to practice development: findings from the literature analysis. *Practice Development in Health Care*, **6**(1), 22–55.

Using this approach had two effects for the team of health visitors, district nurses, school nurses, nursery nurses and community development workers. It ensured proactive community engagement in health improvement and it became a vehicle for developing a public health team. Here is the team's shared vision: 'An integrated team that works in partnership with local communities to build a healthier future for all.' The team had a history of developing innovative projects that benefited community health in their local area, and the motivation for developing the PDU was born out of this. All team members are actively engaged and involved in the PDU, and, through a devolved leadership approach, they have been given the confidence and skills to develop ideas and initiatives that tackle local health priorities. The PDU's journey has been seen as an affirmation of its innovative approach to improving health over a period of several years. In 2006 the team was accredited as a public health practice development unit. This is the story of their journey.

Central Lancashire PCT, UK

The initial work focused on a detailed HNA of the local area, working with community groups, focus groups, schools and Sure Start, among others, plus working closely with the local neighbourhood management team, which was funded by the Neighbourhood Renewal Fund (NRF). Much of the success in building stronger links with the community was attributed to the role of the community development worker, who had good local networks and excellent networking skills. The main health priorities identified were mental health, lifestyle (diet and exercise), and alcohol misuse – its effects on people and as a wider determinant of health.

Successful work programmes include the provision of fresh fruit at weekly clinics held in the health centre. This was an idea led by a staff nurse from the district nursing team and a nursery nurse from the health-visiting team. The Ribbleton community nursing team considered that the large numbers of patients who attended every week were a captive audience for health promotion. Letters were sent to local supermarkets and each supermarket agreed to provide free fruit each week. This was prepared by the team and served to waiting patients, who could join in quizzes and pick up other five-a-day literature at the same time. This initiative has been running for three years.

The team has a strong partnership to develop a local alcohol strategy with community members, licensees, schools and other statutory and voluntary agencies. This innovative approach won an award from the Queen's Nursing Institute to develop and assess a tool for brief interventions. All team members have been trained to carry out brief interventions in minimising harm through alcohol consumption, and this is the basis of their contribution to the strategy.

Project developments are not ad hoc; they are assessed in the development stage for aims, planned outcomes, sustainability and evaluation. If a development receives the go-ahead, it is written into the team's business plan and agreed by a multi-agency steering group. The local university belongs to the steering group that develops clinical practice and theory. The team has become adept at evaluating initiatives and projects as they unfold. All initiatives are based on the HNA and the existing evidence for practice.

The PDU in this integrated team provides a robust model of public health community practice. It is based on a strong and devolved leadership approach to ensure sustainability and maximise shared knowledge and skills. Using evidence-based practice, all projects have a strong element of community engagement. It has strengthened relationships with local community groups using properly evaluated services based on need. The work plan is consistent with the identified health needs, and care is delivered in a variety of community venues by staff with a broad mix of skills. This successful and fully engaged approach to public health care is being rolled out across all the integrated teams in the locality, as it embodies the key elements of modern and responsive health-care services (Kiddy 2007).

In reality there are no quick fixes for the health challenges in many communities. Nevertheless, the key principles and approaches of project development, skilfully and carefully applied, can make a real impact where it matters (Page 2007).

Leading public health practice

Effective leadership is required for many of the public health initiatives in this chapter. There is insufficient room for a long discussion of the evidence and debate on leadership in general and nursing leadership in particular, so here are a few aspects relevant to public health leadership. Kouzes and Posner (2007) have identified five core practices:

- **Leaders challenge the process** – they search out challenging opportunities to change, grow, innovate and improve. Public health is currently high on the government policy agenda and there are huge opportunities to introduce new ways of working, think outside the box and do things differently.

- **Leaders inspire a shared vision** – they see what is possible and persuade others to engage in a shared vision. Winning hearts and minds is a large part of being able to develop public health practice and deliver successful initiatives.

- **Leaders enable others to act** – they do this by facilitating skill development, providing support and offering challenges. They empower people and encourage choice. They promote collaboration and build trust, essential elements of public health practice. They communicate the part each person will play.

- **Leaders model the way** – they set examples and role-model behaviour that demonstrates and supports shared values. Public health leadership is also about being brave and that means having the evidence, believing the evidence, devising solutions and delivering the intended outcome.

- **Leaders encourage the heart** – they recognise individual contributions to the success of every project and regularly celebrate achievement.

Reflective activity

Take some time to think about Kouzes and Posner's five core practices of effective leadership. For each core practice, list two things you already do that help you to be an effective leader. Identify one more thing you could do to make you an even more effective leader.

☞ Keywords

Purposeful leadership
Combines an ability to create a vision in a rapidly changing health service, an ability to motivate people and lead them through change, and an ability to develop innovative ways of delivering services and introducing new ways of working

Purposeful leadership

McNichol and Hamer (2007) have developed a three-dimensional approach to **purposeful leadership** that is also particularly useful in a more practical sense (Figure 9.2). They suggest that the connecting sides of the triangle represent three crucial interdependent elements. The model suggests that any significant shift in any element will have significant consequences for the others. For example, if you increase understanding of yourself, that is likely to increase your capacity to support patient- or client-centred care and contribute to effective teamwork.

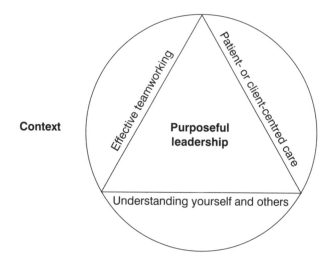

Figure 9.2 Purposeful leadership. Adapted from McNichol and Hamer (2007)

Patient- or client-centred care is about considering the values, preferences and needs of individuals. It is based on the premise that patients or clients know better than anyone else about their health. If they feel empowered, they are more likely to take control of and responsibility for their own health. This is also a central tenet of public health nursing.

Effective teamworking is essential as teams are the building blocks of all organisations. Research into teamwork in the NHS (Borrill *et al.* 2002) has demonstrated some positive outcomes for patients, clients and staff. Health-care teams that function effectively provide higher-quality care, introduce more innovations and save lives. An effective team will have a shared vision, clear objectives, supportive networks and effective leadership. Each team member will know their role and will have their unique contribution acknowledged. Chapter 7 clearly demonstrated the need for partnership working in public health, so it is vital to lead an effective team to engage with the community and other people.

Understanding ourselves and others

To be effective public health leaders, we need to understand ourselves. This can be achieved by reflection, being open to feedback, self-assessment or 360° appraisal (McNichol 2007). Whichever method or combination of methods we choose, the aim is to understand how others see us. This will help us become more effective at influencing and communicating with others, an essential skill in contemporary public health nursing. We must be able to impart a wide variety of complex information to a large population of patients, clients, agencies, professionals and the media. A key skill is the ability to assemble reports or presentations to suit a diverse audience.

Key points **Top tips**

- Start with a bang. If your opening doesn't grab their attention, they won't pay attention
- Write as you speak. Write as if you are talking articulately and knowledgably to another person. Use plain English and don't talk down to the reader
- Put at least one 'you' in your first few sentences, so your reader will feel connected
- Use a variety of methods. People think in different ways: some like facts, some like numbers, and some like logic and detail. Others need the big picture and want to participate
- Break up text with headings, highlight key quotations and summarise the main ideas in bullet points

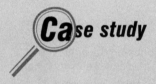
Case study

Anna shows leadership

Anna, a public health nurse, has recently become the leader of a community health team on a housing estate in south-east England. The area is dogged by crime, poverty, alcohol and substance misuse, and there is conflict between groups. It is the last place on earth that people want to be housed. The residents view the health and social care workers as interfering busybodies. Team morale is very low and many of them see no point in working with this community.

Team members experience a lot of stress-related illness, the average burnout time is two years and there is rapid staff turnover. Inexperienced health workers often cover long-term sickness. A variety of services are provided but they are neither planned nor coordinated, let alone effective. Staff work in isolation on individual agendas and keep their heads down. The picture is one of desperation and divisiveness. Here are the stark issues: negative assumptions about people living in these circumstances, lack of direction and engagement, a waste of talent and skills, and demotivation among staff.

- What do you think Anna should do to address the issues? To help you answer, use the three elements of purposeful leadership: patient- or client-centred care, effective teamworking, and understanding yourself and others.
- How could Anna engage people and persuade them to change?

Conclusion

This chapter explained how public health nurses lead and develop practice to improve the health of people, groups and communities. We included the examples to inspire you to join the public health crusade. To develop public health practice you need to create a shared vision, lead an effective team, understand yourself and communicate with others. There are many challenges and the future is uncertain but exciting. Seize the moment and make public health part of everyone's business.

ᴿᴿᴿᴿ**Rapid recap**

Check your progress so far by working through each of the following questions.

1.   What are the seven steps to success?
2.   List the five core practices of leadership.
3.   What are the key attributes of purposeful leadership?
4.   List the three elements of practice development.

If you have difficulty with more than one of the questions, read through the section again to refresh your understanding before moving on.

References

Bar-On, R. and Parker, J. (2000) *The Handbook of Emotional Intelligence*. Jossey Bass, New York.

Benoit, C., Carroll, D. and Chaudry, M. (2003) In search of a healing place: Aboriginal women in Vancouver's Downtown Eastside. *Social Science Medicine*, **56**(4), 821–833.

Borrill, C. S., Carletta, J., Carter, A., Dawson, J. F., Garrod, S., Rees, A., Richard, A., Shapiro, D. and West, M. (2002) *The Effectiveness of Health Care Teams in the National Health Service*. Aston Centre for Health Service Organisation Research, Birmingham.

Castells, M. (2000) *End of Millennium*, 2nd edn. Blackwell, London.

Department of Health (1998) *Signposts for Success in Commissioning and Providing Health Services for People with Learning Disabilities*. HMSO, London.

Department of Health (1999) *Once A Day*. HMSO, London.

Department of Health (2001) *Valuing People: A New Strategy for Learning Disability for the 21st Century*. HMSO, London.

Department of Health (2003) *Building on the Best: Choice, Responsiveness and Equity in the NHS*. HMSO, London.

Department of Health (2004) *Choosing Health: Making Healthy Choices Easier*. HMSO, London.

Department of Health (2005) *Supporting People with Long-Term Conditions: Liberating the Talents of Nurses Who Care for People with Long-Term Conditions*. HMSO, London.

Department of Human Services (Victoria Government Australia) (2007) www.dhs.vic.au/complexclients.

Goleman, D. (1995) *Emotional Intelligence*. Bantam, New York.

Goleman, D. (1998) *Working with Emotional Intelligence*. Bantam, New York.

Harrison, S. and Berry, L. (2006) Valuing people: health visiting and people with learning disabilities. *Community Practitioner*, **79**(2), 56–59.

Kiddy, M. (2007) Public health and practice development. Unpublished report, Ribbleton PDU, Central Lancashire.

Kouzes, J. M. and Posner, B. Z. (2007) *The Leadership Challenge*, 4th edn. Jossey Bass, San Francisco.

McCormack, B., Wright, J., Dewar, B., Harvey, G. and Ballantine, K. (2007) A realist synthesis of evidence relating to practice development: findings from the literature analysis. *Practice Development in Health Care*, **6**(1), 22–55.

McNichol, E. (2007) Understanding yourself as a leader. In: *Leadership and Management: A 3-Dimensional Approach* (eds McNichol, E. and Hamer, S.). Nelson Thornes, Cheltenham, Glos.

McNichol, E. and Hamer, S. (2007) *Leadership and Management: A 3-Dimensional Approach*. Nelson Thornes, Cheltenham, Glos.

McQueen, A. (2004) Emotional intelligence in nursing work. *Journal of Advanced Nursing*; **47**(1), 101–108.

Mencap (2004) *Treat Me Right: Better Healthcare for People with a Learning Disability*. Mencap, London.

Mendoza, F. S. and Fuentes-Afflick, E. (1999) Latino children's health and the family–community health promotion model. *Western Journal of Medicine*, **170**, 85–92.

Page, S. (2007) Editorial. *Practice Development in Health Care*, **6**(1), 1–2.

Salovey, P. and Mayer, H. (1990) Emotional intelligence. *Imagination, Cognition and Personality*, **9**, 185–211.

Social Exclusion Unit (2004) *Breaking the Cycle: Taking Stock of Progress and Priorities for the Future*. HMSO, London.

Strock, M. (2004) *Autism Spectrum Disorders (Pervasive Developmental Disorders)*. NIH-04-5511, National Institute of Health, Bethesda MD.

Thornton, C. (1999) Effective health care for people with learning disabilities: a formal carers' perspective. *Journal of Psychiatric and Mental Health Nursing*, **6**, 383–390.

Totterdell, B. (2004) The practice development accreditation programme at the University of Leeds. *Practice Development in Health Care*, **3**(3), 130–142.

Wright, N. M. J. and Tompkins, C. N. E. (2006) How can health services effectively meet the health needs of homeless people? *British Journal of General Practice*, **56**(525), 286–293.

Young, F. W. (2006) Social problems: a focus for a new branch of public health? *Social Theory and Health*, **4**(3), 264–274.

Appendix: Rapid recap answers

Chapter 1

1. What are the five common causes of death in recent years?

In recent years, the five common causes of death are circulatory diseases, cancer, respiratory diseases, infectious diseases, injury and poisoning.

2. What are the four main eras of public health development?

The four main eras of public health development are the environmental era, the personal preventive era, the therapeutic era and the new public health era.

3. What are the four target areas in the White Paper *Saving Lives*?

The four target areas in the White Paper *Saving Lives* are heart disease and stroke, accidents, cancer and mental health.

4. What are the six target areas in the White Paper *Choosing Health*?

The six target areas in *Choosing Health* are reducing the numbers of people who smoke, reducing obesity and improving diet and nutrition, increasing exercise, encouraging and supporting sensible drinking, improving sexual health and improving mental health.

Chapter 2

1. What are the main principles of public health practice?

The main principles of public health practice are working within a biomedical and social model of health; working within the domains of health protection, health promotion and the maintenance or restoration of health; working with the health and well-being of individuals and communities; working in collaboration and partnership; working with inequalities; working to strengthen communities through the concepts of social capital, social cohesion and social inclusion; and working with healthy public policy and upstream and downstream strategies.

2. What is meant by a community?

In public health terms, a community has a much wider meaning than just a geographical area. It can mean a place where people gather for work, education, worship, social activity or illness.

3. How might a public health practitioner gather information about the health of a community?

A public health practitioner might gather information about the health of a community by carrying out a health needs assessment.

4. How can the area where a family lives affect the family's health?

The area where a family lives can affect the family's health if it is contaminated or polluted directly from local factories, if it has no open spaces for exercise, if it has a high crime rate which makes people feel unsafe to be out and about, if it has a very busy road, if has few shops and they sell fresh food of dubious quality at high prices, if it has poor public transport to good supermarkets, if it has poor schools where young people leave with few qualifications and unable to get a job.

Chapter 3

1. What are the similarities between general nursing practice and public health practice?

The similarities between general nursing practice and public health practice are assessing need, planning priorities, implementing interventions, and evaluation.

2. Name the three main models of public health practice.

The three main models of public health practice are preventive, participatory and political.

3. List three core skills that are common to public health practice and nursing or health-care practice.

Three core skills are communication skills, interpersonal skills and therapeutic intervention skills.

4. List five generic public health skills.

Choose any five from these generic skills: assessing needs, partnership work, prevention or minimisation of harm, raising awareness, project working, implementing policy, enabling, leading and managing, evidence-based practice, managing ethically and effectively.

Chapter 4

1. What are the four types of need?

The four types of need are felt, expressed, normative and comparative.

2. How does a sociologist's perspective of need differ from an epidemiologist's?

A sociologist views need as closely related to social factors such as poverty, unemployment, housing and education. An epidemiologist is interested in data on the amount of disease in a population and the associated risks and number of deaths.

3. What are the key perspectives of HNA?

The key perspectives of HNA are the epidemiological perspective, the sociological perspective, the economic perspective and the consumer perspective.

4. Identify three purposes of HNA.

Choose any three from these HNA purposes: search for and raise awareness of needs; identify the pattern of health and illness and health inequality; set priorities, influence policies or target unmet needs; plan appropriate interventions and services; enable efficient and effective ways of using resources to maximise the benefits of health care.

5. What five steps help to ensure a comprehensive HNA that results in action?

Here are the five steps: (1) get started by asking

questions about the population, what you want to achieve, who needs to be involved and what resources are required; (2) identify health needs and priorities; (3) assess a health priority for action; (4) plan a public health project; (5) conduct a review.

Chapter 5

1. Name the data you would use to measure health.

Data you would use to measure health are quantitative data such as epidemiological data (mortality, morbidity, prevalence, incidence) and hospital data (admissions, discharges, waiting lists), and qualitative data such as views from professionals, views from the public and the knowledge in the community.

2. What can demographic data tell you?

Demographic data can tell you about population size, population distribution and population characteristics such as age, gender, ethnic group, religion, socio-economic status and deprivation score.

3. What four factors should you consider when appraising data?

Check that the data is accurate, timely, complete and valid.

4. What tool is needed to appraise the evidence for public health interventions?

Use the Critical Appraisal Skills Programme (CASP) to appraise evidence for public health interventions.

5. What is the difference between validity and reliability?

Validity is about whether evidence is accepted or approved as the truth. Reliability is about whether evidence is accurate and representative and whether it can be replicated.

Chapter 6

1. Explain the difference between health promotion and health education.

Health education is one aspect of health promotion; it tends to focus on one person at a time and gives them information on how they can improve their health and start to change their behaviour. Health promotion is a wider concept that covers a range of activities.

2. **What are health beliefs?**

   Health beliefs are factors that influence the actions a person takes with regard to their health.

3. **Define the three levels of health promotion.**

   Primary: healthy people are empowered to follow a healthy lifestyle and to use preventive services. Secondary: people who have an illness or disease are helped to recognise the impact of unhealthy behaviour and to seek a remedy. Tertiary: people with a long-term condition are encouraged to participate in rehabilitation and to change their lifestyle to promote independence.

4. **List and define the different approaches to health promotion.**

   Educational: to develop knowledge and skills that enable an informed choice. Medical: absences from disease. Behavioural: individual decisions to change behaviour in a specified way. Client-centred: working with clients to establish their goals either individually or as a community. Social: create physical and social environments that promote a healthy lifestyle.

5. **Identify models for health promotion practice.**

   Some models for health promotion practice are the health action model, the health belief model, the stages of change model and the theory of reasoned action. The purpose of using a health promotion model is to help plan a programme and to link theory to practice.

6. **What activities are most useful to help people change their behaviour?**

   Activities that are most useful to help people change their behaviour are activities that improve self-esteem, confidence and assertiveness. They may include individual and group work such as skills training, advice and education. They may also include the wider elements of health promotion, such as displays, campaigns and using mass media.

Chapter 7

1. **List three potential outcomes of a good partnership.**

   Choose any three from these potential outcomes: solutions to problems that single agencies cannot resolve, promoting citizen involvement, better coordination of services across organisational boundaries, avoidance of duplication, and making best use of available resources.

2. **Name three characteristics that define a high-quality partnership.**

   Choose any three from these characteristics: common aims and a shared problem, an agreed plan of action, mutual respect and a cooperative relationship, good communication, creativity, risk taking, shared responsibility.

3. **Identify the key drivers that underpin the shift towards integrated working.**

   Partnership working is being driven by international and national public health policy plus changes in legislation from central government; appreciation of the wider determinants of health and growing support for population-based core public health functions; the recognition of complex health needs that cannot be met entirely by a single agency; economic imperatives that mean a single agency cannot afford to fund a project on its own; common commitment to a project so that no single agency bears sole responsibility.

4. **What are the key steps in making partnership work?**

   These are some of the key steps in making a partnership work: establish a working relationship through good communication skills and processes; seek to promote mutual understanding and gain consensus through ground rules; agree goals and working procedures that enable all parties to make a full contribution; be creative and agree to celebrate diversity; promote collective ownership to include collective responsibility for success and failure; record and evaluate progress and achievements.

Chapter 8

1. **What is outcome evaluation?**

   Outcome evaluation evaluates what has been achieved, the end result.

2. **What is process evaluation?**

   Process evaluation evaluates how the end result was achieved by examining whether the most efficient approach was used to deliver the end result.

3. **What are the purposes of evaluation?**

   The purposes of evaluation are to determine effectiveness, to develop a knowledge base, to improve a service, and to demonstrate cost-effectiveness.

4. **List five approaches that can be used for evaluation.**

   Choose any five from these approaches: randomised controlled trials (RCTs), questionnaires, statistical analysis of data, interviews, informal feedback, direct observation, and reflection.

5. **Why is goal setting so important for evaluation?**

   Goal setting is so important because the goals determine what must be measured to test whether the intervention has been successful.

Chapter 9

1. **What are the seven steps to success?**

   The seven steps to success are (1) engage people; (2) be community leaders; (3) be service leaders;
   (4) deliver care in a community-based framework; (5) make links with the growing community resource networks; (6) make links with regional, national and international colleagues; (7) give priority to high-risk groups.

2. **List the five core practices of leadership.**

   Leaders challenge the process, inspire a shared vision, enable others to act, model the way and encourage the heart.

3. **What are the key attributes of purposeful leadership?**

   The key attributes of purposeful leadership are effective teamworking, a patient- or client-centred approach, and understanding yourself.

4. **List the three elements of practice development.**

   The three elements of practice development are quality improvement, evidence-based practice, and creativity and innovation.

HILS

Health Information and
Library Service
Gateshead
Primary Care Trust

Index

Page numbers in *italics* indicate figures, tables or boxes.